Modern Myths and Medical Consumerism

The Asclepius Complex

Antonio Karim Lanfranchi

Translated by Jonathan Hunt

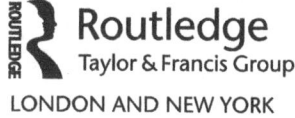

Routledge
Taylor & Francis Group

LONDON AND NEW YORK

First published 2018 by Routledge

2 Park Square, Milton Park, Abingdon, Oxfordshire OX14 4RN

52 Vanderbilt Avenue, New York, NY 10017

Routledge is an imprint of the Taylor & Francis Group, an informa business

First issued in paperback 2019

Published in Italian by Moretti & Vitali in 2010 as *La vita appesa a un filo. Miti d'oggi e consumismo sanitario.*

Translated by Jonathan Hunt

British Library Cataloguing-in-Publication Data
A catalogue record for this book is available from the British Library

Library of Congress Cataloging-in-Publication Data
Names: Lanfranchi, Antonio, author.
Title: Modern myths and medical consumerism : the Asclepius complex / Antonio Lanfranchi.
Description: Milton Park, Abingdon, Oxon ; New York, NY : Routledge, 2018. | Includes bibliographical references.
Identifiers: LCCN 2017056721 (print) | LCCN 2017059060 (ebook) | ISBN 9781351167642 (E-book) | ISBN 9780815348221 (hbk) | ISBN 9781351167642 (ebk)
Subjects: LCSH: Medicine—Philosophy. | Physician and patient.
Classification: LCC R723 (ebook) | LCC R723 .L348 2018 (print) | DDC 610.1—dc23
LC record available at https://lccn.loc.gov/2017056721

ISBN: 978-0-8153-4822-1 (hbk)
ISBN: 978-0-367-40827-5 (pbk)

Typeset in Sabon
by Apex CoVantage, LLC

Modern Myths and Medical Consumerism

Modern Myths and Medical Consumerism is concerned with the loss of a sense of limit in technological medicine today, and the way in which the denial of death leads to an uncontrollable, consumeristic multiplication of needs. Taking its starting point from C. G. Jung's analytical psychology, the book gives a symbolic interpretation based on archetypal, philosophical and socio-psychoanalytic ideas developed through the author's personal experience, moving from the medical to the psychoanalytical paradigm.

Lanfranchi depicts ideal sources of medicine, based on archetypal material drawn from Greek myth, and discusses the progressive steps of the doctor's consciousness' evolution up to contemporary times. Critiquing current medicine and its 'modern myths', the book suggests the prevailing model of economic development is unsustainable, and provides prospects of a more contained ecological medicine and an ethical approach that will allow readers to reflect and move towards a more qualified attitude to mortality.

The book meets the need to transform medicine into a critical domain of human experience, capable of providing essential services consistent with the naturalness of death and environmental sustainability. As such, it will be vital reading to academics in the fields of psychotherapy, analytical psychology, psychiatry and medicine, and those with a philosophical or sociological background.

Antonio Karim Lanfranchi is Senior Cardiology Specialist at the University Hospital L. Sacco, Milan.

Research in Analytical Psychology and Jungian Studies Series

Series Advisor: Andrew Samuels
Professor of Analytical Psychology, Essex University, UK

The *Research in Analytical Psychology and Jungian Studies* series features research-focused volumes involving qualitative and quantitative research, historical/archival research, theoretical developments, heuristic research, grounded theory, narrative approaches, collaborative research, practitioner-led research, and self-study. The series also includes focused works by clinical practitioners, and provides new research informed explorations of the work of C. G. Jung that will appeal to researchers, academics, and scholars alike.

Books in this series:

Jung and Kierkegaard
Researching a Kindred Spirit in the Shadows
Amy Cook

Consciousness in Jung and Patañjali
Leanne Whitney

Shame and the Making of Art
A Depth Psychological Perspective
Deborah E. Cluff

Modern Myths and Medical Consumerism
The Asclepius Complex
Antonio Karim Lanfranchi

For more information about this series please visit: www.routledge.com/Research-in-Analytical-Psychology-and-Jungian-Studies/book-series/JUNGIANSTUDIES.

To Cristina, Edoardo and Guglielmo

Contents

Figures

Acknowledgements

I wish to thank Luigi Zoja, whose constant intellectual stimulation was essential for the realization of this project. Thanks also for the support of Eva Pattis, Enrico Moretti and Carla Stroppa. Feelings of gratitude go to friends and colleagues, Paolo Bergmann, Philip Bechtel, Massimo Lemma, Evangelos Tsempelis, Alessandra Di Montezemolo, Giovanni Sorge, Donatella Buonassisi and Roberto Grande, who were helpful in different ways during the writing process. A special acknowledgment to my mother, Sania Sharawi Lanfranchi, and to my sister, Mariangela Soraya Lanfranchi, for their continuous intellectual and material assistance. My gratitude also goes to the Teachers and Colleagues of the C. G. Jung Institute, Küsnacht, Zürich. Finally my most heartfelt gratitude goes to my wife, Cristina, for her joyful presence and unending conversation, and to my sons, Edoardo and Guglielmo, to whom this book is dedicated.

Introduction

On Attic stelae, did not the circumspection of human gesture amaze you?
Were not love and farewell so lightly laid upon shoulders, they seemed
to be made of other stuff than with us? Oh, think of the hands, how they
rest without pressure, though power is there in the torsos. The wisdom of
those self-masters was this: hitherto it's us; ours is to touch one another
like this; the gods may press more strongly upon us. But that is the gods'
affair. If only we too could discover some pure, contained narrow, human,
own little strip of orchard in between river and rock! For our heart transcends us just as it did those others. And we can no longer gaze after it
into figures that soothe it, or godlike bodies, wherein it achieves a grander
restraint.

—Rainer Maria Rilke[1]

One of the most common concerns of doctors in large hospitals and health
organizations is that of 'being forced to work with numbers' rather than
people. The demand for productivity and the limited time allotted by administrators to each task limits the doctor's relationship with the patient to the
dehumanizing uniformity of automatisms of a technical nature.[2] There is
a proliferation of 'normative' procedures intended to promote the correct
application of scientific and organizational protocols, under the reassuring umbrella of 'guidelines'. Doctors submit to the constant pressure to do
things, sometimes abandoning any attempt to think, to reflect; believing
that they are free, they in fact have great difficulty in providing an autonomous basis for their freedom. At the same time they become complicit in the
economic power and mystificatory projections associated with science. The
supra-personal role of doctors who place themselves above their patients,
indulging their own projections, is accepted in the name of a higher reason,
a metaphysical belief in science, contrary to the true scientific spirit. This
allows doctors and health organizations to embody the extraordinary power
of technology in their own persons, to become the instruments of its histo-
ricization in the tissues of the human body, rational agents of an absolute,

self-sufficient evolution. A totalitarianism of the techno-scientific machine results in moral compromise; a host of often unnecessary surgical and therapeutic procedures are deterministically accepted and normalized, raising the spectre of systemic waste and unsustainability.

The principle of reality is now the uncontested domain of technological uniformity; we seem to be living in a glorious new Promethean age, which is equipped with the latest technology but newly unaware, for the pace of technological evolution is much faster than that of the individual consciousness.[3] Having discovered the new technological fire, human beings are carried away by the exercise of the power that it brings with it, and by the predominance of quantity over quality. Any ethic apart from that of productivity is demoted to a subordinate rank, and it becomes more difficult to put into practice an ethic of responsibility, or indeed to adopt any kind of ethical position. Moreover, communication between doctor and patient is impeded by the very nature of the technological factor and by the vast gap in knowledge created by an increasing specialization. The cognitive divide is the counterpart of technological efficiency. Technology separates knowledge, and can obstruct individual awareness as a process.

In health organizations, too, there seems to be a split between, on the one hand, the conscious attitude, based on objectifying reason, supported by the idea of growth and concretized in the dogma of accumulation and profit, and, on the other, the menacing spectre of unsustainability, of the finiteness of resources, which tends to be ignored and repressed. But the underlying cause, at both poles of the doctor-patient relationship, is probably an unconscious denial of the insuperable limit of life, namely death, the greatest taboo of contemporary humankind.

The discussion in this book will show how the *repression* of death becomes an object of commercial exploitation, of a creation of the superfluous. Moreover, the prescribed treatment, intended to restore individuals to a condition where they can function properly in society, clashes with unconscious psychic factors of a personal and collective nature, which are consequences of the living complexity of reality, in which many people ignore their own limits, thus intensifying the already widespread cultural and emotional alienation.

The constant pressure to rationalize organizational and managerial methods is an attempt to direct, limit or 'govern' a paradoxical demand for health, whose irrational origins lie beyond the sphere of intervention of the administrators of the health organizations themselves. The recourse to concepts such as 'governance', 'risk management' and what is termed 'evidence-based medicine' seems like a *deus ex machina* designed to replace with logical surrogates the sense of extraneousness to the problem. Moreover, scientific research in the medical field is one-sidedly directed towards the development of new ways of treating illness and thereby postponing the prospect of death. Consequently it is a generator of costs, as this is the only field where the virtuous link between technological development and investment indirectly translates into a further economic deficit, because of the ever-increasing age of the treated population, the creation of a wide range of patients suffering from multiple chronic conditions, and the exploitation of a welfare system which has difficulty in organizing itself, precisely because of the failure to find a solution to these paradoxes. The extent of expenditure on healthcare and of the accompanying 'systemic waste' threaten the historical prospect of a universal right to health; consequently, technological civilization betrays its Enlightenment roots by not actively confronting the problem of the finiteness of human life.

It is to be hoped, therefore, that doctors and patients will re-examine the paradigm by which health problems are approached. A freer vision is needed, one which includes in its decision-making processes a knowledge of the various kinds of unconscious conditioning and of the forms of behaviour that derive from them, not only at the individual but also at the collective level.

The narrative takes its inspiration from these themes, drawing principally on my own inner psychic reality, based on my personal experience as a cardiologist in several public hospitals in Milan. I have tried to provide a key to the psychological and symbolic interpretation of the ways in which my colleagues and I relate to each other and to others, both in the clinical practice of medicine and in the non-material sphere of our work. The writing of this book has been like repeating the same journey many times over, with the aim of developing a humanistic sensibility in the doctor's consciousness.

The doctor's mask, or 'persona', is a powerful shield in the dominant culture; in our collective consciousness it is associated with dedication, willpower, precision, self-sacrifice, tenacity, competence and study – all qualities which can easily determine different degrees of identification of the ego with the persona (or role identity). One-sided extroversion, or the split between the outer dimension, often characterized by a stern superego, and the inner one, which is often ignored and repressed, can become a source of profound alienation in this difficult profession.[4] If at one extreme of the spectrum there are personalities which are one-sided, because they strongly identify with their role, at the other there are more sensitive individuals, who experience more consciously the tension, not only on the objective, professional level but also on the inner one, between the need for self-representation and the need to confer meaning. As is well known, in the medical profession cases of somatization, addiction (notably to work, food, alcohol and other drugs), occupational disease and burn-out are very frequent. For all these reasons, a conscious experience of the relationship between doctors, paramedics and patients may generate an authentic, meaningful sphere of interpersonal exchange, more capable of imposing limits, and at the same time compensating for the needs created by the technological spirit of our age.

Written at a time of change on both the personal and professional levels, this book brings together three main voices from my experience as a doctor and a human being. The first is the mythic-symbolic voice, a sort of 'thinking in images', an inner invention which interweaves themes, some personal, some more general, and which attempts to trace their archetypal sources, sketching out a meta-psychological history of medicine. Sources of inspiration for this sometimes rather hermetic voice are Karl Kerényi's *Asklepios*[5] and, more generally, James Hillman.[6] Alongside this voice runs a narrative voice inspired by my direct experience with patients. Lastly, the third voice is that of more abstract reasoning, or 'psycho-social' interpretation, always in dialectic tension with the other two. In the effort to harmonize these three voices, I have chosen to make it my primary task to convey a not yet fully formed concept of responsibility and global human solidarity, leaving the fundamental questions open, so that my readers themselves can search for possible answers.

Notes

1 Rilke 1923, pp. 37, 39.
2 See, for example, the epigraph at the beginning of this book. Levi 1947, p. 152.
3 See Jaspers 1949, pp. 112–126: 'Misjudgements of the limits of technology' and 'Perception of the demonism of technology'.
4 On psychic reality, on the Jungian concept of *persona*, on splitting (for the splitting of the ego and for the splitting of the object), on the superego, see Laplanche and Pontalis 1973.
5 See Kerényi 1948.
6 Hillman, several works, see following chapters.

Bibliography

Jaspers, Karl (1949), *Vom Ursprung und Ziel der Geschichte. The Origin and Goal of History*, translated by Michael Bullock, New Haven & London: Yale University Press, 1953.

Kerényi, Karl (1948), *Der göttliche Arzt: Studien über Asklepios und seine Kultstätten. Asklepios. Archetypal Image of the Physician's Existence*, Bollingen Series, Vol. LXV.3, New York: Pantheon Books, 1959.

Laplanche, Jean & Pontalis, Jean-Bertrand (1973), *The Language of Psycho-Analysis*, with an introduction by Daniel Lagache, translated by Donald Nicholson-Smith, London: Hogarth Press, 1973.

Levi, Primo (1947), *Se questo è un uomo*, Turin: Einaudi, 1958.

Rilke, Rainer Maria (1923), *Duiniser Elegien. Duino Elegies*, The German text with an English translation, introduction and commentary by James Blair Leishman and Stephen Spender, Third Edition (revised), London: The Hogarth Press, 1948.

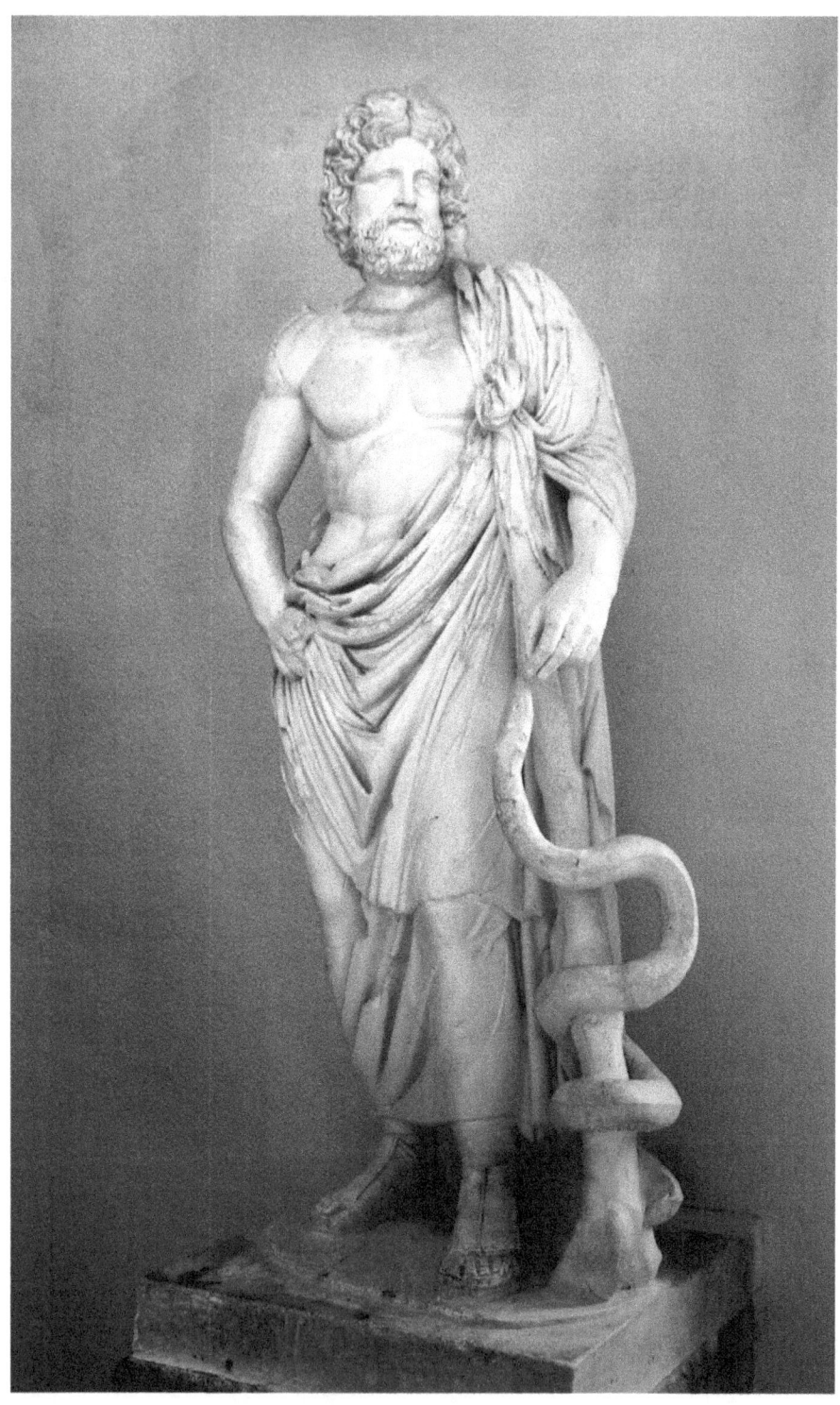

Figure 0.1 Asclepius, with his serpent-entwined staff. Archaeological Museum of Epidaurus.

© Michael F. Mehnert – Wikimedia Commons.

Part I

A metapsychology of the doctor's consciousness

Chapter 1

The story of Asclepius

The birth of Asclepius and the symbolic origins of medicine

In Greek and Roman mythology, Apollo had the power not only to cure human diseases and wounds, but also to inflict them. On the one hand he was the solar principle of life and knowledge, the basis of order and symmetry, god of the arts, medicine, music and prophecy. On the other hand he could strike at the human world anywhere with his unerring bow, and was therefore the 'cause' of all sickness and pestilence. According to a Roman oracle, only he who had caused a disease had the power to cure it, and that was Apollo himself. Medicine, therefore, is a quintessentially Apollonian art.

Apollo the physician was the father of Asclepius. The story of the latter's birth is told in Ovid's *Metamorphoses*. Asclepius was born of Apollo's love for Coronis, a mortal woman of royal blood. Apollo fell in love with her when he saw her bathing on the shore of a lake in Thessaly. After they had consummated their passion, he left the crow, whose feathers were white at the time, to watch over her. Soon afterwards, encouraged by her father Phlegyas, king of the Lapiths, Coronis married Ischys. The crow flew to Apollo to tell him about it. The god was so furious that he turned the bird's plumage black to punish it for not keeping Ischys away from Coronis, and the colour has characterized all its descendants to this day.

Apollo knew that Coronis was already carrying his child. In a fit of rage, he picked up his bow to punish her for her betrayal. As soon as he had released the arrow he realized the folly of his action, but it was too late, for an arrow fired by a god can never miss its target. Guilt frequently precedes action in this way, being already present in the intention; the thinnest of threads prevents a thought from being immediately turned into action. When the tension becomes uncontrollable, the thread can release the accumulated energy, resulting in a rash act whose consequences are both unpredictable and irremediable.

Overcome with grief and remorse, Apollo ran to embrace the woman he still loved, and she died in his arms. To atone for his guilt, he laid her body on the funeral pyre, as ritual required; it was a heinous offence not to honour the dead. But as the fire burned, he cut from her womb the baby – his son Asclepius, the god of medicine.

Coronis's fate was sealed by the violence of the male members of her family. Her fate illustrates femininity's lack of autonomy with respect to an archaic male principle, and its coercion by that principle. The situation goes back far earlier than the events that culminated in Asclepius's birth. The violent history of the menfolk of Coronis's family links Asclepius's human origins to the dark, fiery, hellish side of nature.

Asclepius's mother came from a cursed lineage. Her father Phlegyas tried to burn down the temple of Apollo in Delphi. His name recalls the Greek verb *phlego* and the Latin verb *flagro*, both meaning 'to set fire to', or 'to burn'. It is emblematic of sudden, blazing anger, a dark, smouldering fire that is always ready to flare up. His story would make him the perfect ferryman for the Styx in Dante's *Divine Comedy*.

His son, Ixion, Coronis's brother, killed his guest Deioneus in a particularly cruel manner, by tricking him into falling into a pit full of burning coals. Ixion tried to rape Hera, the queen of the Gods, and was punished by being tied to one of the wheels of the sun's chariot. His relationship with Nephele was said to have given rise to the race of the Centaurs.

The Centaurs themselves were subject to violent, uncontrolled outbursts of rage when drunk on wine. They represent the violence of the pre-paternal male group, whose characteristics are coercion and an animalesque, warlike inebriation unmitigated by any feminine charm. The only way the group can relate to women is through lust, possession and rape.[1] Significantly, a descendant of this line was the wise Chiron, himself a centaur, the first physician and Asclepius's teacher.

Phlegyas and Ixion represent the destructive violence of fire, the untamed, terrifying nature of the pre-technological age, against which the human race struggled from prehistoric times until the discovery of fire and the first technological, or Promethean, era.[2] According to Kerényi,[3] Coronis's husband Ischys represents Apollo's 'dark double', and in particular his destructive side – the urge to destroy which is inherent in Asclepius's genealogy. So the transformation of fire into the funeral pyre lit by Apollo's love and repentance is striking. Asclepius is born from that fire. Apollo's action, in snatching his son from his mother's burning womb, suggests a paternal desire for reconciliation with a feminine principle of mercy and grace, in contrast to the violent, uncharitable nature of the male members of Coronis's family. The father's reparatory gesture brings forth a divine child, enriched by the events that had accompanied his conception and birth. Indeed, the child's birth, according to Kerényi,[4] was in fact a rebirth, in the sense that one side of Apollo's nature emerged to replace another: a lethal power was transformed into a healing one. Later Asclepius's hubris proved his downfall: he was burned to ashes by one of Zeus's thunderbolts for daring to substitute his omnipotence for nature. Asclepius dies because he is unable to conquer the element – death – which characterizes not only his destiny but also his art and knowledge.

Symbolically these events shape Asclepius's art of medicine. On the one hand he embodies the solar principle inherited from his father Apollo, the agent of life. On the other hand, paradoxically, he embodies the 'hidden fire' inherent in the violent potential of human nature – a fire that destroys, rather than providing light. But the 'hidden fire' also implies a possibility of redemption. It will cease to be hidden when Prometheus steals it from the gods and gives it to man. As a result, fire is transformed and tamed; it can be used by humankind, becoming an incarnation of *techne* in matter.

The Apollonian keenness of Asclepius's gaze, according to Kerényi,[5] is tempered by a sadder, warmer tint – a tragic shade, suggesting affinities with Dionysus. Wine played an important part in ceremonial sacrifices to the 'physician-god', too. The proximity of the Asklepieion, or temple of Asclepius, to the theatre of Dionysus in Athens, and of the tomb of the *heros iatros* (health-bringing hero) to the shrine of Dionysus at Marathon, indicate a link between Asclepius and Dionysus. Asclepius is born from Coronis's ashes, just as Dionysus is born from the ashes of Semele, daughter of Cadmus and Harmonia. Semele fell into a trap set by the jealous Hera. Pretending to be her friend, Hera instilled in her a desire to be united with Zeus in his divine form, knowing that this would result in her death. The king of the gods tried in vain to dissuade her, but eventually, compelled to do so by a promise, he appeared to her in all his splendour, burning her to ashes. This seems to be a metaphor for divine inebriation, and for the mad god who would be born. Zeus saved the child that Semele bore in her womb by sewing it into one of his thighs, where it completed its gestation.[6]

Both Asclepius and Dionysus, then, are characterized by a special link, from birth, with the dimensions of fire and death; both are born from a dying, or 'burning', womb: in one case consumed by a human, earthly fire lit by the god, in the other burned to ashes by the fire inherent in Zeus's divine nature. Dionysus, however, must continue to mature in his father's thigh – he has not completed his gestation; unlike Asclepius, he is not yet completely 'born'. The symbolic meaning of the link between these two gods and their cults will be discussed later (p. 97).

Asclepius possesses an innate sensibility that will develop into a knowledge of human suffering, in a borderland between life and death, represented by his symbolic animals, the serpent and the dog. They stand for the natural, chthonian and emotional aspects of the human being.

Sick people would spend a night in the temple, in the protected space of the *temenos* ('sacred precinct', from *temno*, to cut, split). The two animals would appear to them in a dream, in the likeness of handsome young men bearing the gift of healing. Sometimes the god himself would appear as a divine child. Illness was experienced as a process of initiation; after initial purification, the sick person would be sent into the sacred protected space inside the Asklepieion and there be bitten by the serpent, thus having a symbolic experience of death. This would be accompanied by a theophany, or encounter with the god in a dream. The person would be reborn into a human condition enriched with sensibility and knowledge because of the transition that had occurred – or, in psychological terms, because of their integration of an unconscious content.

Protected by the ritual container of tradition, individuals do not shrink from this experience, but participate in the process of healing, preserving their links to the vital energies (of the unconscious). They do not merely 'undergo', and are not merely 'patients' (from *pathos*, to suffer). So they are not absolutely distinct from a healthy person. On the contrary, the initiate/patient actively integrates both conscious and unconscious content, (re)constructing their identity in a fertile exchange with the temple/world outside. There is no clear distinction, but only a symbolic gradient, between health and sickness.

In our own time, this experience is subject to the principle of causality inherent in medical science. That science has to make appropriate changes to the process of the disease in order to achieve 'recovery'. In the *temenos*, the experience becomes an inner experience situated on the threshold of the communicable, on a terrain different from that of science – namely the individual's own capacity for symbolization. Individuals are not patients, but people who 'incubate' the possibility of their own evolution – that is, already contain that evolution within themselves, protecting it and cultivating it, by the intercession of the god. The outcome of that evolution is not 'causally' predetermined. In this sense there are similarities with the process of *individuation*, 'becoming oneself', which in analytical psychology takes the place of the clinical concept of healing.

In his *Attempt at Self-Criticism*, Nietzsche says of his *Birth of Tragedy* that it is 'constructed of nought but precocious, unripened self-experiences, all of which lay close to the threshold of the communicable, based on the groundwork of art – for the problem of science cannot be discerned on the groundwork of science.'[7]

In the same way it may be said of modern medicine that only by standing outside the field of clinical scientific reasoning can we hope to identify the underlying problem of medicine. If we do not include within our thinking a symbolic view, centred on our relationship with the patient, we lose the most significant dimension of the experience of illness, and the potential deriving from the patient's particular world view (*Weltanschauung*). The Cartesian distinction between subject and object which underlies the principle of causality in scientific explanatory medicine leads us to express all knowledge according to the dictates of objectifying reason. This approach seems reductive, however, with respect to the psyche's own way of knowing things, which operates on several different levels simultaneously – the rational, the emotional, the symbolic and the sensorial. However useful to science the distinction between subject and object, soul and body (or psyche and soma) may be, in the experience of major events like illness it becomes arbitrary. A transitional area is created in the patient's inner experience – a far more vaguely defined and constantly changing area, but a crucially important one, for it expresses its particular dimension, the uniqueness of its limit and therefore the unrepeatability of its approach to death. This condition of liminality, which does not fall within the field of reality of every scientific hypothesis, can, if it is included and properly exploited in the patient's relationship with the doctor, become a potential source of knowledge for both parties. In the *temenos* it lies at the centre of the therapeutic process.

Asclepius's childhood, from Chiron to Prometheus

For his education and upbringing Asclepius's father entrusted him to the care of the centaur Chiron, the son of Cronus (Saturn to the Romans) and Philyra (Figure 1.1). The latter, in a version of the myth reported by Kerényi, was so alarmed at the sight of her new-born son that she turned herself into a lime-tree.[8] The figure of Chiron is hybrid in every respect: he is both animal and vegetable, solar and chthonian, divine and human, refined and wise but at the same time endowed with the violent disposition of the centaurs. This chimerical being lies at the origin of the founding principles of ancient medicine and symbolizes the centrality of a contradictory and polar knowledge of nature, the way it stands up to the tension of its origin and its survival despite all opposites, in particular the infinite sphere of the inorganic, to which life is destined to return by an innate and ineluctable predisposition.

Chiron, the first physician, significantly introduces Asclepius to the secret properties of matter and the knowledge of medicinal plants, the first *pharmaka*. For ancient pharmacology, the boundary between curative action and toxicity is not only a quantitative question, but is also linked to a traditional knowledge and an initiatory context. The taking of the *pharmakon* occurs

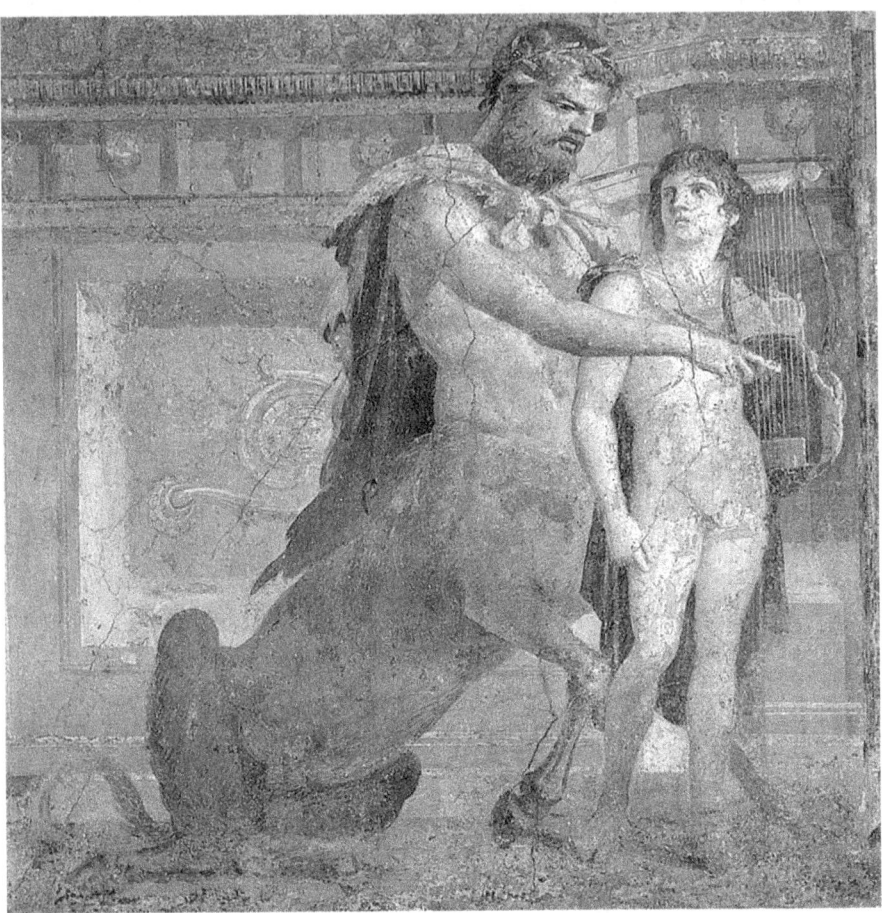

Figure 1.1 Chiron instructs young Achilles. National Archaeological Museum, Naples, Italy. Unknown photographer – Wikimedia Commons.

in a ritual dimension, the container of the curative process (in contrast to the modern prescription of medicines, which is at risk of repetitive and consumeristic degeneration).

A medicine is natural poison and as such recalls the serpent, which from Asclepius's childhood onwards always accompanies him in the vicinity of the cave where he was brought up. Coiled around his wand, it will become the symbol of medicine, sometimes confused with the caduceus (the rod carried by Hermes, or Mercury), which is derived from the ancient Greek *kerykeion*, from *keryx*, a 'herald'.[9] The serpent lived, figuratively or actually, in special recesses within the *temenos* of temples, and, as Jung indicates in *Symbols of Transformation*,[10] it expresses its meaning on several levels. In the first place it is a symbol of the richness of instinctual life. From here it branches out into two contrasting meanings: like the dog, which Jung associates with Hecate and Anubis, it becomes a symbol of death as well as of life. So the serpent's well in the temple of Cos was also the 'treasure house', into which the faithful dropped coins through a crack or slot in the ground. The serpents were the 'guardians of the treasure' – of the threshold between the two kingdoms, the container of the precious hoard of which patients must gain possession and 'take with them' on re-emerging from their sleep in the *temenos*. Significantly, Chiron's home, a cave at the top of Mount Pelium, is also a doorway into Hades, surrounded by a vast garden of medicinal plants.

The theme of retrieving the treasure brings us to the myth of the hero and to what I consider to be one of the essential features of the doctor's identity. For the treasure one has to recover is life itself. 'The treasure which the hero fetches from the dark cavern is life: it is himself, new-born from the dark maternal cave of the unconscious where he was stranded by the introversion or regression of libido.'[11]

The serpent is one of the most spiritual of all creatures. It is, according to Jung,

> both toxic and prophylactic, equally a symbol of the good and bad daemon (the Agathodaemon), of Christ and the devil. [. . .] It is an excellent symbol for the unconscious, perfectly expressing the latter's sudden and unexpected manifestations, its painful and dangerous intervention in our affairs, and *its* frightening effects.[12]

It indicates the fear of (mortal) regression to the mother's womb, as a symbol of the eternal cycle of death and rebirth; the mother who only generates and only destroys, devouring the children she herself generated. The dark side of the feminine and of a poorly differentiated male conscience is emphasized here. But this very fear takes on a fundamental function, that of protection and the impulse towards making the most of life. The individual, as in the initiatory mythology of the hero, will have to do one of two things: either overcome the apathy induced by the serpent's bite, shaking off the sleep of childhood and dependence on adult life and rising to the level of his or her potential; or, if these things have already been achieved, move away from the peak and accept the path of decline and return, which is indispensable to the renewal of life. If it is conscious, this movement becomes voluntary transformation and maturation rather than submission to the dominance of fate or surprise in the face of the inevitability of loss.

According to Jung, if we do not accept the risk of facing up to fear, the meaning of life will be in some way violated.[13] Moreover, this death is not our external enemy, it is our own 'inner longing for the stillness and profound peace of all-knowing non-existence, for all-seeing sleep in the ocean of coming-to-be and passing away.'[14]

It is therefore in a particular dynamism and its changes, both in a progressive and in a regressive direction, situated between the extremes and extremisms of life and death, that the psychic or symbolic experience of death resides. We will see later how the mythologem of the hero, so closely linked to the fear of the feminine, conditions both the need for systematic denial/repression[15] of all vulnerability and the supreme domination over matter that is characteristic of modern medicine.

The greatest expert in medicines, Chiron, is pierced, accidentally or in fulfilment of the decree of destiny, by an arrow steeped in the most terrible poison, that of the Hydra. Hercules had fired the arrow at the centaur Elatus, but it went on to hit Chiron, who had also been his former master and teacher. There is no antidote for the poison. So the quintessential hero, a symbol of light and consciousness, is the unintentional but fatal destroyer of Chiron's ancient chimerical wisdom. Unable to die, for he too is a god, Chiron lives in the most atrocious torment, which he is powerless to relieve; the great expert in herbs and poisons finds himself in the paradoxical position of not being able to save himself. Chiron's existence is therefore marked, like that of every human being, by an eternal closeness to suffering, but, according to a metapsychological interpretation, also by the inevitability of the decline of his ancient wisdom in the face of the rise of the heroic world of humankind. He must renounce his immortality to escape the terrible pain to which he is condemned; with this image, the encounter with pain becomes a presupposition of *individuation* for the human being: Chiron being forced by the reality of his pain to give up his immortality. It seems to be no coincidence that, in exchange for his death, Zeus agrees to put an end to the suffering of Prometheus, who had been freed from his chains by Hercules, the solar hero of iron will and rationality. Zeus accepts Chiron's death in exchange for the liberation of Prometheus, and transforms Chiron from a present reality close to humanity into a celestial deity, the constellation of the Centaur, to be contemplated in the distance. Chiron's sacrifice elevates humanity, which has long forgotten its ancient natural wisdom. He gives it the gift of the fire of knowledge, *but separates it from any profound symbolic identification with nature*. This is perhaps the origin of the modern repression of pain and death, the temptation to entrust its 'management' to the aseptic hands of *techne*. Note the analogy with the symbol of original sin, where the fall of man follows his eating the fruit of the tree of knowledge.

It is understandable, then, that Greek thought, from Pindar onwards, abandoned those archaic figures of primordial mythology, characterized by profound ambivalence; Pindar considered Chiron a dead god. He represents the end of ancient medicine and its heroic evolution with the advent of technological medicine.

The Asklepieions and the medical tradition[16]

The Homeric tradition did not regard Asclepius as a god, but as a hero, an excellent doctor who had become the object of a cult in later generations. According to Homer, only Paean, the physician of the gods, could be divine, personifying the epiphany of life in the process of healing. But it is only in the world of the gods that he can manifest himself in the pure and total state.

Mortals, by contrast, merited the skill of a great physician, who certainly did not possess such ethereal power. Nevertheless, the miracle of every cure was celebrated by humankind with invocations and songs which testified to the god's presence. He was often invoked in his capacity as a divine child, symbolizing the mysterious and vital regeneration inherent in recovery. In this there was a quality that derived from the patient's own nature, something outside the physician's sphere of control. At the crucial moment, something comparable to a wellspring is activated, and its water flows through the patient, originating from the god yet at the same time representing a link with the depths of the earth; significantly it was an essential feature of Asklepieions that they should contain a spring of water. The *temenos* inside the Asklepieion serves both to mark out the sacred space and to give it life. It was the crucial place in the temple, where patients would spend the night, waiting to be visited in their dreams by the god (*incubatio*), often in the form of a handsome young man (the dream, as was mentioned earlier, was the oneiric equivalent of the serpent's bite). The *temenos* represents the container of the space of healing, a boundary inside which gifts were offered, a small sacrifice was made, in something resembling a 'slot' or a 'door', thus acting out the separation and, at the same time, the equally real conjunction between one thing and the other and therefore between the self and the other person. The patient was separated from the external world, entering a space of transition and expectation, which alluded to its vital centre, and in which the patient found a 'new' body. In psychological terms, it was a sacred precinct which had the functions of protecting and guarding, but at the same time acting out the split parts of the personality safely in the consciousness, as if on a stage. In this protected space – a container created by trust, under the guidance of the physician/teacher – the individual is able to draw on the wellsprings, the place of inaccessible physical and psychic energy, to re-emerge renewed, not lapsing into fusion with the undifferentiated or primordial world (*mater*, mother/matter).

Only a sick person – not the parturient or the dying – could be admitted to the temples of Asclepius. Moreover, the Hippocratic writings required anyone wishing to practice medicine to consider the teacher as a father. There was no charge for the teaching, and the pupil became in effect a 'brother' of the teacher's natural children. All doctors, or Asclepiads, considered themselves descendants of the god. The transmission of medical teaching followed two different but interlinked traditions: first, that of the *religio medici*, linked to the cult, symbols and images of the god; second, a *techne* – knowledge and skill handed down as family tradition and hereditary talent. With the advent of modern medicine, these traditions were abandoned in favour of technical manipulation, which is detached and reifying. But by objectualizing nature, one loses the symbolic understanding of it (*habentibus symbolum facilis transitus est*, 'transition is easy for those who have a symbol', ran an old alchemical saying) and the mystery of the relationship with the patient no longer occupies a central position.

Beyond Prometheus: the end of tragedy and the coming of dialectic – the rational origins of medicine

The abandonment of tradition with the rise of technological medicine could be symbolically represented by the liberation of Prometheus, as is suggested by the equivalence between fire and technology. It originates from the seminal change in the mentality of the Greeks with the advent of Socratism and the historicizing of humankind. The true break with the mythical past lies in the optimistic subversion of the tragic spirit of the Greeks by dialectic and by the serenity of the dying Socrates, whose heart conceals the secret conviction, as Nietzsche states in *The Birth of Tragedy*, that science is able not only to reach the centre of being but actually to change or correct it:

> a profound *illusion* which first came to the world in the person of Socrates, the imperturbable belief that, by means of the clue of causality, thinking reaches to the deepest abysses of being, and that thinking is able not only to perceive being but even *to correct it*. This sublime metaphysical illusion is added as an instinct to science and again and again leads the latter to its limits.[17]

In this deep-seated conviction we see the myth that is inherent in science. Significantly, during his trial Socrates repeatedly states his belief that he has a divine vocation and (like Descartes) finds it necessary to create a *deus ex machina*, to justify the determinism of reason. At his death, he tells those present not to be sad, and his last words refer to Asclepius: 'Crito, we owe a cock to Asclepius. Don't neglect to give it to him.'[18]

It seems that Socrates, in thanking Asclepius, after the 'arguments' in favour of the immortality of the soul presented in the *Phaedo*, was emphasizing the sublime achievement – rational serenity, even in the face of death. This may explain the possible irony of his phrase, mingled with the bitterness of the hemlock. According to Hillman, Socrates was stressing, in his very last moments, that

> once the cocky pride of life that crows hopefully at each day's dawning is sacrificed, the instinct for tomorrow is yielded. Death then is the cure and the salvation and not just a last, worst stage of a disease. The cock crow at dawn also heralds resurrection of the light. But the victory over disease and the new day begins only when the ambition for it has been abandoned upon the altar. The disease which the experience of death cures is the rage to live.[19]

It might be said that Socrates's last utterance in a sense redeems the egoic breadth of his work.

Nietzsche writes again in *The Birth of Tragedy*, 'The presupposition of the Promethean myth is the transcendent value which a naive humanity attach to fire as the true palladium of every ascending culture.'[20] Prometheus's original sin is an active sin, which becomes virtue, the price of which is always the suffering inherent in the human condition, after the theft of knowledge from the sphere of the divine. 'Man, elevating himself to the rank of the Titans, acquires his culture by his own efforts, and compels the gods to unite with him, because in his self-sufficient wisdom he has their existence and their limits in his hand.'[21]

With Prometheus, man becomes able to 'take upon himself' the fire of contradiction inherent in the heart of being. His knowledge is not devoid of tragic awareness, it has not yet become one-sided. The titanism of Promethean man does not, therefore, arouse *phthonos* (the envy of the gods), because, 'with the heroic effort made by the individual for universality', it does not deny 'the misery in the essence of things';[22] it knows that in life cruelty is inseparable from happiness, it knows the immanence of death in the arc of life, and knows that for every individual, death is total, not generative, that it cancels once and for all the oneness of every person. It is the discovery of the naturalness of death that drives man to learn to reify and dominate nature. It is the first disenchantment in history or, we might say, the first disenchantment from which the very possibility of history originates. The fundamental shift in organized civilization with the coming of Prometheus is indispensable to the beginning of the axial time of reason, historical time.[23]

As Salvatore Natoli points out, with Prometheus,

> the living in general (*physis*), and human beings in particular, tend to push death away by becoming provident. [. . .] The original antagonism of life and death takes on a new figure in civilized humanity; such human beings feel that they have a right to dispose and dominate [the universe that surrounds them], and therefore feel free to kill. In this way they become provident and warlike.

They 'begin to construct their existence, and so guard and develop it.' Human beings learn from Prometheus 'the contrast between technology and necessity; they learn in their effort the impossibility of becoming gods, and at the same time the arrogant expectation that they will become gods.'[24]

With the coming of the axial time of history, if human beings push away the spirit off the earth so as to be able to reify the world and dominate it, they experience an age of transition, that tension between irreconcilables which constitutes existence. At the same time, they arm themselves and become wary of the prospect of death, which, though invincible, is at least kept at a distance, by affirming and protecting the fullness of living. The development of a reason detached from nature, starting with Socrates, Plato and Aristotle and culminating in the atomic bomb, becomes the creed of the human race's progressive technological domination over nature.

The collectivity of human beings organized in increasingly global social structures takes over nature's role of dominating the individual, and appropriates the natural instance of destruction, once a divine faculty, which affirms life, and, in so doing, kills.

But from this position, *homo artifex*, who is able to take action and foresee things, while not denying the tragic tension between opposing necessities presided over by Dionysus (the god of laceration and dismemberment), remains constantly at risk of hubris. Inflation tends to rise again, with the intention of alleviating pain, from the constant propensity to the illusion of happiness and to the unconscious temptation to emancipate the self from death, a temptation of power which had always been inherent in the nature which humankind has appropriated. This tendency becomes predominant and Narcissistic in present-day global capitalism, with the new fire of energy (understood as power) and information technology.

However – to return to Nietzsche – a higher justice, reigning over human beings and gods, derives from the intuition of the encounter between

Promethean-Dionysian laceration and the spirit of art, the dominion of Apollo, and delimits the lust for life, giving man the 'splendid deception'. This magnificent illusion of an encounter, the matrix of the myth, gives musical, aesthetic form to the joy of transcending the fundamental dissonance of being, without denying it. The intuition of the intimate union of music with myth, of a beauty that does not praise the hero for his victories but raises him, emphasizing his ruin and defeat (like that of Oedipus at Colonus), shines in his tragic view of the world; its point of departure is not detachment or renunciation, but a peculiar kind of emotion, very different from the pathos of the theatrical style of modernity, being based on the acceptance of caducity and chance. The intuition of the encounter between Dionysus and Apollo, of the intimate link between their two natures, in the possibility of a unitary vision of the world, gives life to the symbol, which is ultimately nothing else but the tragic myth itself. The art of medicine feeds on this link, which brings us back to the close relationship between Asclepius and Dionysus.

Today, the metaphysical illusion of science, strengthening the conviction that causality can penetrate the abysses of being and correct them, has the crucial effect of countering the fear of death in an individual consciousness that has existed for only a few centuries, and of making existence seem comprehensible and therefore justified. Socrates the mystagogue of science becomes the founding hero of the needs of a bourgeois humanity, which will triumph in history by pursuing its magnificent illusion.

This digression shows that it is the rise of what might be termed Socratic medicine, even more than that of the Promethean variety, that removes the tragic vision and eliminates the pessimism and sense of limit that are inherent in the very heart of Greek culture. The separation between art and science, beauty and justice, begins here. Later, with the coming of Christian monotheism, it will prefer to hide the 'terrible face' of God behind a veil, until it arrives, in a secular manner, at its denial. At this point the flowering of the scientific spirit becomes possible, and it is perhaps here that the intrapsychic reality of death starts being denied and the initiatory nature of the processes of treatment begins to be lost.

With the coming of the modern age, humankind will endeavour to forget the lesson of wise Silenus, Dionysus's teacher and follower. Captured by King Midas after a long chase through a wood, he was forced to answer the question, what was the best and most desirable thing for humankind:

> Oh, wretched race of a day, children of chance and misery, why do ye compel me to say to you what it were most expedient for you not to hear? What is best of all is for ever beyond your reach: not to be born, not to *be*, to be *nothing*. The second best for you, however, is soon to die.[25]

Silenus was an ugly, deformed satyr, who, like Pan and Chiron, represents closeness to instinct and the precious wisdom that derives from it, the basis of the tragic spirit of the western world.

Nourished by all these events, Asclepius grows up knowing how his teacher died and how Prometheus was set free. The race of centaurs descended from his uncle Ixion, so Asclepius is acquainted with their violent, impulsive nature. The essence of the centaur, as a symbol of male violence, is rape, combined with the warlike impulse of the band of soldiers, which indicates 'a regression of maleness to the animal herd and the physical strength deriving from numbers.'[26] The myths about centaurs allude to the instability of the civil condition, to its interspersion with the animal condition and with the realm of instinct. For Ixion was conceived without *charis*: without the benediction of the Graces – that is, without feminine grace or a loving relationship. His life, and that of his descendants, would be marked by this double absence. But Chiron is the exception that indicates that preserving the relationship with animal nature (the man joined to the horse) is therefore an occasion of disorder but also of knowledge. So Asclepius is able to know, as a result of his education by Chiron, the profound ambivalences of nature. By contrast, Hercules, the prototype of the hero, is unable to have a dialogue with the male element most closely linked to instinct (the centaur, which is half animal): 'he can only *poison it and repress it*; in so doing, he kills its most creative elements (Chiron and Pholus).'[27]

Since he has no dialogue with instinct, the unextinguished germs of animal ferocity will persist in him in a repressed form. The Herculean world of the rational will, of purposeful attention, will have to carve out new balances and contain new tensions, and those balances are always threatened by this violent impulse, in organizations, for example, or in hospital hierarchies. The risk of a return of repressed violence will continue to hide behind the strictness of patriarchal hierarchies which admit of no vulnerability, and in the intricacies of secular rationalism which prolongs life, offering worldliness and the destruction of myth in exchange for safety.

Nature personified: Pan

At every spring, as James Hillman says, there is a nymph,[28] and this brings us to Pan: the nymph represents the object of desire, the anima, the complement of instinctual male coercion. In her the brutality of instinct finds an intrinsic possibility of 'reflection', on the imaginal level. Every wellspring was personified, so the fount of the *temenos* was too. Pan's death had been announced by Plutarch in *The Twilight of the Oracles*. The nymphs were 'personifications of the wisps and clouds of mist clinging to valleys, mountainsides, and water-sources, veiling the waters and dancing over them,'[29] as is confirmed by Homer in the *Odyssey*.

'In every nymph there is a Pan, in every Pan a nymph. Rawness and shyness go together.'[30] Pan, the goat-god, was loved by all the gods, and particularly by Dionysus. The song of this solitary goat was the origin of tragedy (etymologically derived from *tragos*, the male goat). Associated with ravines, forests, dark caverns and precipices, he represents nature personified and animated; he is both the material recess of desire, as in the neo-Platonic tradition, and the horror associated with the coercions of instinctual nature. Pan and the nymphs are as one, two poles of the same archetype, indicating that the human animal instinct has a capacity for self-reflection quite different from satisfaction and release – instinct self-mitigates within itself and is transformed, gaining a certain degree of freedom. Psychologically, the desire that impels Pan to pursue and the nymphs to flee is linked to rape, nightmare, 'panic' and masturbation: at the very moment of its actualization it is frustrated. From the alienation of desire, a psychic space residual to it is created, and this space is reflected on the impulse of instinct and, above a certain threshold, generating a psychic form, a mental image that is thought to originate from the very heart of living matter. As Jung wrote, in this connection:

> *Reflexio* is a turning inwards, with the result that, instead of an instinctive action, there ensues a succession of derivative contents or states which may be termed reflection or deliberation. Thus in place of the compulsive act there appears a certain degree of freedom. [. . .] Through the reflective instinct, the stimulus is more or less wholly transformed into a psychic content, that is, it becomes an experience: a natural process is transformed into a conscious content. Reflection is the cultural instinct *par excellence*.[31]

Pan's loves are mythic representations of this process; their multiplicity reveals the initial impersonality and fluctuation of desire, which later settles into a definite path. Pitys is a nymph of the fir tree. Syrinx is a Naiad who escapes his sexual assault by metamorphosis (this is a later tradition, reported by Ovid), turning into a reed from which Pan made his pipes, the most direct example of the transformation of nature into culture. The incorporeal Echo frustrates Pan's desire, in a more direct symbolic expression of the concept of *reflexio*. Eupheme, 'the politely spoken one', is the nurse of the Muses, whose gentle use of words nourishes art by renaming and ennobling the god. Selene, the moon goddess, whose conquest induces Pan to hide his hairy black parts under a white fleece, is a symbol of whitening that reflects the feminine light of the moon, like a torch blazing in the night. All these women were loved by Pan, and each of them gives instinct with a chance to reflect itself inside itself and therefore to 'see' by means of desire, thus reclaiming compulsive projection as imagination.[32] This innate ability to generate images is the origin of the compensatory function of dreams in analytical psychology, and establishes the link between the conscious attitude and the creative nature of the unconscious. So the fact that Asclepius's epiphanies occurred in personified form in dreams may be seen as a gift from Pan to the art of medicine. 'The person of Pan the mediator, like an ether who invisibly enveloped all natural things with personal meaning,'[33] made possible the epiphany of his meeting with the wounded healer, Asclepius, in sickness, as in every other natural process.

The death of Pan, the end of personified nature, marks the beginning of the reification of nature and of the body's vicissitudes. Each natural 'object' ceases to speak to us; disease becomes attribute or property, symptom and sign, medical semiotics. Pan ceases to be a support and orientation of Psyche, the expression of a delicate wisdom which derives from the body and expresses the reliability of instinctual life, as in the story told by Apuleius.[34] And in this way nature can be 'controlled by the will of the new God, man, modelled in the image of Prometheus or Hercules, creating from it and polluting in it without a troubled conscience.'[35]

Prometheus, in challenging the gods, encounters suffering commensurate with the weight of the burden he takes upon himself, which had formerly been projected on to the gods. After stealing fire from the gods, he will always find himself, in every new enterprise, at risk of inflation. The enrichment of consciousness with a new unconscious content 'swells' the ego and makes necessary a difficult work of integration. It does not seem to be a coincidence that the Dionysus Zagreus of the mystery rites is torn apart by the Titans, Prometheus's brothers, representing the sacrifice of symbolic knowledge and the risk of a return of the repressed which this involves. This also includes the fact that the repressed may either be projected on to the other, or, alternatively, fall into the soma, attacking the body. The opposites move apart and at the height of the conflict the tension becomes excessive: the neuro-vegetative imbalance induces a somatic illness, a 'rash', a hypertensive crisis, a fibrillation, a colic, a reflux, a headache, a 'fainting fit'.

The risk of the modern perspective, when it becomes one-sided, is that it may not be limited to the denial of the archetype/symbol, but may actually cause the *splitting* of its two fundamental polarities:

> As the human loses personal connection with a personified nature and personified instinct, the image of Pan and the image of the Devil merge. Pan never died, say many commentators on Plutarch, he was repressed. Therefore, [. . .] Pan still lives, and not merely in the literary imagination. He lives in the repressed which returns, in the psychopathologies

of instinct which assert themselves [. . .] primarily in the nightmare and its associated erotic, demonic, and panic qualities.[36]

If the repressed Pan becomes the devil, the nymphs become witches; the feminine is concretized and deprived of its imaginal dew. Its image may be perverted, as when the feminine is reduced to a doll, sexualized and objectualized, or into the distorted, punitive, menacing version of the feminine which competes and deprives instead of nourishing.

Pan returns not just as a symptom, but also as an archetypal shadow, absolute evil, which merges with the dark colour of the Germanic Wotan. He becomes a collective shadow in the age of the great repression of natural death; repressed death will be projected on to the other and it will be possible to treat it with the indifference of a one-sided consciousness dissociated from instinct and from the community of destiny in the face of which instinct makes us equal. The goat becomes a scapegoat. Other people's dead become less pitiable, they are no longer even moving, for they are distant.

Pan also becomes the devaluation of life in favour of artifice, a prevalence of the laws of the market over the value of human experience. This might be the origin of the mercantile shade of medicine – medical finance – and its limiting idea of humanity, where the individual doctor too often ends up replacing ethics with the 'labels' of the pure reductive approach to nature.

In the same way, when the polarities of the archetype of knowledge and life – the Apollonian and the Dionysian – separate, the splits between science and art, justice and beauty, ideal and real, abstraction and common sense – splits which are the cause of such confusion and moral indifference in the contemporary world – reappear. There is a return to the central problem of psychology – what is inauthentic? – in an age where the crowd seems to have become the condition of all authenticity; as Jaspers says in *Genius and Madness*, referring to Hölderlin and Van Gogh, what is authentic is the profundity in which the ego destroys itself, the hypertrophic and abstract ego of modernity, which is compelled to see the authentic only in its own destruction, and to acknowledge an awareness of the divine presence only in the mentally ill.[37]

The fragmentation of both archetypes points towards the antinomic separation between nature and culture: in the one case here on earth, in the other in the lower heaven of Olympus. In the first case, it will strip the earth and hide it under a cloak of ignorance and artifice; in the second, it will drive heaven so far away as to make it invisible and inaccessible.

The Asclepius complex: the descent and death of the god

In the Homeric age, doctors were also warriors: Asclepius's sons were first and foremost the leaders of the Thessalian contingent in Troy: Machaon, the first surgeon, and Podaleirius, who could heal 'invisible' maladies, including those of the soul. There is no mention in the *Iliad* of the third son, Telesphorus, the 'bringer to completion' (of the process of convalescence); a dwarf, he assisted his father. Asclepius's wife, Epione, was the goddess of pain relief. Their daughters were Panacea, the goddess of universal healing through plants and the Mercurial spirit of the rod; Hygieia, the goddess of prevention and the personification of health; Iaso, the goddess of convalescence, the personification of healing; Aegle, the goddess of natural beauty and mother of the Graces; Aceso, who presided over the healing of wounds; and Meditrina, the Roman goddess of health, longevity and wine. In classical representations, Asclepius's daughters often appear together with a serpent.

The root of the name Machaon is *mache*, battle, expressing the unity in his person of the doctor and the warrior. Machaon was wounded in the Trojan War by Eurypylus, he of the 'wide gate', indicating his relationship with the infernal dimension of the medical art: wounding and being wounded are the dark premise of healing; they made the medical profession possible and are essential to human existence. Every wound can be healed, but a human being as a whole cannot, and will ultimately prove mortal. Machaon, indeed, dies in battle, but is survived by the cult associated with him, that of a hero who wounds, heals and is himself mortally wounded. The link between wounding and healing in Machaon expresses the direct link with the action characteristic of the surgeon; the warlike spirit does not yield to fatalism, and in this is a precursor of the technological manipulation of nature inherent in modern medicine.

Asclepius, too, is associated with the underworld: according to Hesiod's account, he was condemned to death by Zeus for bringing Hippolytus back to life and thereby contravening the divine law of the Fates; Zeus struck him down with a thunderbolt and consigned him to Hades for ever. This expresses an intuition of the risk of *inflation*, the development of a sense of omnipotence, which crosses the boundaries of death, when it imagines that it can not only heal wounds, but symbolically redeem the whole individual from death. The physician's sense of omnipotence might be described as an *Asclepius complex*, deriving from identification with a superhuman power of life and death and the consequent psychic inflation. According to the myth, when Asclepius was at the bedside of the dead Glaucus, a serpent came and coiled around his rod. Asclepius killed it, whereupon another serpent arrived and restored it to life by feeding it with the leaves of an herb. Asclepius used the same herb to bring

Glaucus back to life, and others after him. So the physician's power complex was the reason why Zeus burned Asclepius to ashes with thunderbolts made by the Cyclopes, whom Apollo then killed in revenge.

The refusal to accept the boundary between life and death, and the determination to redeem life by denying death, has its roots in the origin of the medical art. The surgeon, a modern warrior, who makes use of technology, risks losing the veil of humanity that is present in Asclepius's vision, thus moving away from the patient towards the 'higher' Apollonian one-sidedness, which does not see death and suffering. This is a risk well known to many surgeons – the good ones – who understand when it is right for them to stop.

It is interesting to note, in this connection, that in other versions of the myth, both Chiron and Asclepius are taken up into the heavens after death and turned into constellations, the Centaur and Ophiucus, the serpent-carrier. Their divine status is restored to them, this time forever, but as a result they move away from the world of modern technological humanity, leaving a fertile field to the spirit of Prometheus and that of Socrates.

Chiron and unrepressed death

A tree sinks its roots into the earth while aspiring to the sky; it feeds on the depths and is transformed, turning towards the light. In the mind, the tree is a symbol of the self, a bridge between the primordial parents after their separation. It comprises both the depths of the abyss and the seed's struggle towards the surface, towards the separation of consciousness and differentiation. The harmonic tension that links its terrestrial and celestial parts in a continual creative act expresses the function of *centroversion*, which Neumann describes as the natural tension – between the call of one's origins and the struggle for knowledge – to take up a position on the axis of the personality mid-way between the realms of the ego and the self, outside the ego but not too far away from it.[38]

If trees express presence and silent contemplation, the imperious recall of the vegetable kingdom and reassuring proximity, in this they are different from the animal instinct, whose desire, exploration and constant questing we more easily feel, alternating with the epiphanies of instinctual coercion. Chiron's nature contains a natural, though chimerical, balance between the human element and the animal and vegetable worlds.

Jung writes:

> Whenever the 'simple' and 'kindly' old man appears, it is advisable for heuristic and other reasons to scrutinize the context with some care. [. . .]

> The old man has a wicked aspect too, just as the primitive medicine-man is a healer and helper and also the dreaded concocter of poisons. The very word φάρμακον means 'poison' as well as 'antidote', and poison can in fact be both.[39]

When Chiron is struck by the arrow of Herculean will, which does not distinguish him from the other Centaurs, the drama of the end of an era begins. The Hydra's poison gives him excruciating pain; it is a constriction of the great sage's mind, forcing him to suffer the fate decreed by the hero. Hercules shoots the poisoned arrow perhaps as a result of a *lapsus*, or simply by chance. The Hydra's poison recalls the terrible implementation of the devouring aspect of the great mother, characteristic of solar heroes, not of an old Centaur like Chiron, who is able to accept and at the same time dominate his earthly nature. It is the archaic parts of Hercules, however, not of Chiron, that seem to be projected with the poisoned arrow. He kills the old Centaur, in the same way as Socrates and Euripides kill tragedy. But human beings draw from this will, which dissociates reason from instinct, the strength to direct the consciousness one-sidedly and to make its action clear and direct, on a linear path of history.[40]

Still, Chiron cannot die, and his wealth will not be entirely lost. The human being's natural wisdom cannot die. It is an ever-accessible resource, simultaneously animal and vegetable, and antithetical to the one-sidedness of the hero, consumed as it is by the vital need to overcome attachment to the mother. Ontogenetic and individuative closeness to nature becomes a knowledge of the tensions of Chiron, balanced between the Apollonian world and earthly roots. His world and its tensions are assimilated and transformed in the education of Asclepius, his apprentice and adopted son.

In his essay 'Plato's Pharmacy', Jacques Derrida points out that in the *Phaedrus* the word *pharmakos* is systematically excluded from the significant word-chain *pharmakeus-pharmakon-pharmakeia*, which often recurs in the text.[41] Socrates is the *pharmakeus*, the wizard, sorcerer or poisoner, and shows that sophistic dialectic, in the sense of discourse, is closer to truth – that is, to the primeval world of ideas – than is writing. Reading a written text is seen as imitation, compensation for a *hypomnesis* (re-memoration, recollection, consignation) contrary to the truthful procedure of *mneme* (living, knowing memory), the word that comes directly from the sphere of ideas.[42] For this reason Plato criticized both writing and painting, judging them to be imitative, and therefore inauthentic, arts. In the *Phaedrus* Socrates describes the *pharmakon*, never mentioning its meaning of poison, which alludes to the unspoken word *pharmakos*, a homonym of *pharmakeus*, but at the same time compared to something like a scapegoat. The *pharmakos* was originally an outcast, a repulsive creature, an unfortunate who was first nurtured, then driven out and killed outside the walls in the ritual of the scapegoat. At times of calamity for the social group, evil was externalized and eliminated, though in fact its externality has always been part of the chain of meaning. Consequently, in the ambivalence of the word *pharmakon*, the boundary between destructive and therapeutic action remains a thin one; it always hides a residue of meaning, an inexhaustible fund (*fond sans fond*), a diacritical reserve exceeding every pair of opposites, which constitutes Plato's Pharmacy.

> The ceremony of the *pharmakos* is thus played out on the boundary line between inside and outside, which it has as its function ceaselessly to trace and retrace. *Intra muros/extra muros*. The origin of difference and division, the *pharmakos* represents evil both introjected and projected. Beneficial insofar as he cures – and for that, venerated and cared for – harmful insofar as he incarnates the powers of evil – and for that, feared and treated with caution. Alarming and calming. Sacred and accursed. The conjunction, the *coincidentia oppositorum*, ceaselessly undoes itself in the passage to decision or crisis. The expulsion of the evil or madness restores *sōphrosunē*.[43]

Sophrosyne was the goddess or spirit (*daimon*) of moderation, self-control, temperance, measure and discretion. She was one of the good spirits that escaped from Pandora's vase. Her Roman equivalents are Continentia and Sobrietas.

The *pharmakon* is both poison and drug, but also medicine and cure, and this ambiguity develops on the border between the outside and inside of the chain of meaning. In the experience of the Asklepieions the body becomes a 'subtle body', sacred and significant to the same degree as the natural process and its interaction with herbs and remedies. In this context, the imaginal dimension of the epiphany of the god and the dream is as 'real' as the serpent's bite. Serpents and herbs are constant companions of Asclepius's childhood and life, around the cave where he lives. The god grows up breathing the air of the archaic universe dominated by the chimerical tensions of Chiron, and indeed by one of the gateways into Hades. The gateway into the underworld, as has already been mentioned, might represent unrepressed death, which is central to the beginning of every initiatory process and to every ritual context, and expressed by the experience of pain in illness. This is the death that Hercules and Prometheus – rationality and technology – will try to expel from the world and consciousness 'for ever'.

The double meaning of poison and medicine, then, depends not only on the size of the dose, but also on the context; if the burden of pain is consciously accepted, and the emotional content is processed, the resulting alienation does not generate anger at living, and is not vented in compensatory avidity. So, if the experience of death, and therefore of the personal limit, is not repressed *at the beginning* of the illness, it becomes impossible to know its tension. This leads to the possibility of developing a new mode of consciousness, a meaningful state, which is still, however, obliged to compare within itself the tension of death and rebirth.

If, on the other hand, the process is inverted, as it usually is nowadays – that is, if death, understood as pain or privation, is completely denied – it re-emerges at the end of the process, as a return of what has been repressed.[44] The stimulus represented by the poison or drug (the serpent, the unconscious psychic or somatic content) will be constantly pursued, producing a gradual increase in the 'dose', and therefore addiction. This leads to psychic inflation (an excess of life) alternating with depression (a sense of death, nihilism, as the outcome of the process). On the somatic level, this is equivalent to an alternation between 'unconscious', functional life, the 'clean bill of health' of our medical certificates, and a demonization of disease, which is in fact part of that good health.

The inversion of the initiatory process is one of the causes of the greed and gigantism typical of healthcare consumerism. One example of this on the somatic level is the compulsive eating of seriously overweight individuals; another is the spread of addiction to so-called 'social' drugs (cocaine, alcohol, synthetic drugs), which does not always impair the individual's performance. Often there is no specific individual psychopathological anomaly, but only a passive acquiescence, on the part of more vulnerable subjects, in the collective value of functionalism and consumption, even hyperconsumption. This bulimic tendency, which ultimately becomes self-destructive, is heightened in two ways: in a negative sense by the principal taboo of the dominant culture – the absence of any symbolic representation of death – and in a positive sense by the central value attached to money, with its enormous power constructs. The high-calorie, meat-based diet has been promoted by appealing to these psychological factors, presenting attractive images of well-being which induce people to consume, while repressed death reveals itself in the consumer's self-destruction and in the virtual indifference of business corporations to the environmental sustainability of their policies. The great spread of cattle farms, monocultures and deforestation, all phenomena necessary to supporting the global diffusion of this kind of food, are, as is well known, responsible for biological impoverishment and for most of the greenhouse effect. To this should be added the passiveness of consumers and the capitalist's moral indifference to the huge increase in pathologies linked to this kind of diet, especially heart disease and cancer. In the future, disease itself, not just of the body but also of the mind, will have a compensatory psychological meaning both for the individual and for society. Death will continue to make its presence felt – externally, in environmental devastation, and internally, in the many detrimental effects of overeating. But increased ill health will create a further market for new technological and commercial appetites of a medical kind, creating a vicious circle, which will never end as long as it is supported by a distorted idea of the welfare state – another kind of addiction, but this time supported by society as a whole.

Asclepius's progeny: the breaking up of the archetype[45] and the beginnings of specialization

The death of Asclepius goes hand in hand with the emergence of a structural change in the relationship between consciousness and the unconscious with the coming of modern medicine. However, shifting the libido from the level of 'mystical participation' (*participation mystique*)[46] to that of conscious differentiation and analysis comes at a price: the reduction of the signifying power of the relationship with other people and the impoverishment of the relationship with the extraordinary richness of the unconscious (nature and the 'other' inside us). Though transformed and contained, the domain of instinctual life is controlled and impoverished. Becoming aware of this risk can help to prevent the loss of an essential component of individual potential, on which the possibility of transcending the values of the collective conscience, which begins from the individual, depends.

After Asclepius's death, the process of *differentiation* continues with the fragmentation of his archetype into a number of different principles, represented by his wife and children, which will become specialized fields of medicine. The centrality of the archetype of the wounded healer, inherited from the archaic world of Chiron, is 'broken down' into a variety of elements, which can be more easily accepted by the mind as qualities and specialized areas of medicine. Formerly an art, medicine becomes more and more a science. These elements will continue to revolve around the original nucleus, still represented even today by the Hippocratic oath, but will gradually acquire a *raison d'être* of their own. As was mentioned earlier, while Asclepius remains associated with intensive care, because he brought several patients back to life, Epione becomes a metaphor for anaesthesiology, Hygieia for hygiene and preventive medicine, Panacea for pharmacology,

Aegle for aesthetic medicine and cosmetics, Iaso for rehabilitation, his son Podalirius for physical and mental diagnostics, and Machaon for surgery and, we might add today, interventional therapeutics.

In Greek mythology, Epione, or Epion ('the reliever of pain'), is a nymph. The princess of Kos, also known as 'the Meek one', she becomes Asclepius's wife. As it happens, her name is almost identical to the Greek word for opium – *epion/opion*, or 'juice' – for it is derived from the juice of the poppy and is therefore associated with anaesthesia. The first example of the use of opium as an analgesic came when her sons Machaon and Podalirius treated Philoctetes's wound.

Aceso, the goddess of the healing of wounds and the curing of diseases, represents, unlike her sister Panacea – the process of curing, not the cure itself. Her male counterpart is Telesphorus, he who 'brings to completion' convalescence from illness or wounds, in an active sense. His temple, the *Telesphorion*, is in Pergamum, in Anatolia.

Panacea, the goddess of healing through the use of medicines, herbs and other remedies, is a forerunner of pharmacology. Her shadow might be the charlatanry of the 'universal remedy', which hides, like hope trapped inside Pandora's vase. In the alchemic and Neo-Platonic tradition, Panacea is the spark that can be revived in the heart of being, a universal remedy to free the *anima mundi* imprisoned in matter, but also the *serpens Mercurialis* of Asclepius's rod, a hermetic, imaginal, analogical and metaphorical modality.

Iaso is the personification of health, in the sense of the manifold ways of achieving healing; she seems to be identified with the personal nature of the routes that lead from sickness to health, so she again underlines the importance of personified nature in the process of healing. It is natural to connect her with the individual effort of re-exercising the *functio laesa* peculiar to each patient in the processes of rehabilitation, both on the physical level and, for example, on the neuro-linguistic level, where programmes are personalized and adapted to the individual combination of defects.

Aegle, the goddess of radiant good health, or natural beauty, is described by some writers, including Plutarch, as the daughter of Asclepius and Lampetia, daughter of the Sun, by others as the daughter of Asclepius and Epione. Her name means 'splendour', 'brightness', denoting the beauty and harmony of the human body, when in good health. Aegle's aura is ageless, but is constantly imitated by cosmetics, and by aesthetic medicine and surgery, and is constantly being re-presented in new ways by advertising.

Hygieia, known to the Romans as Salus, is the goddess of good health, a companion of Aphrodite. Sometimes portrayed as a mother, with a calm demeanour, associated with the bud of a plant and with fertility, queen of Apollo, who procreates life and health, and whose will only Hades can resist.[47]

Indeed Apuleius contrasts her with Persephone. But above all, various sources (Aeschylus, Hesiod, Vergil and Seneca) contrast her with the Nosoi, spirits or *daimones* of disease and the plague. Hesiod describes them fleeing from Pandora's vase, while Elpis (hope) remains trapped inside. He represents them as being personified to a certain extent. In most Homeric literature, however, it was the arrows of Apollo and Artemis that brought pestilence. The Roman equivalents of the Nosoi were the Morbi: Lues and Pestis (pestilence), Tabes (emaciation, consumption) and Macies (putrefaction, decay). Algos (Dolor to the Romans), not one of the Nosoi, represents emotional and mental pain, which leads to despair. The Greek Keres, female death-spirits, agents of the Moirai (the Fates), and daughters of the night, were, like the Moirai them-selves and Thanatos, occasional personifications of mortal illness. In classical sculpture, Hygieia is often portrayed with a serpent, which she feeds from a bowl with her own hands. In works of art, a considerable number of which have come down to us, she is represented as a virgin, wearing a long dress, with a kind, gentle expression, a relative of the Graces (Charites), either alone or in the company of her father or her sisters. Although she was originally the goddess of good physical health (what we would call today 'a strong constitu-tion'), she was also seen as the protector of mental health, and so was identi-fied with the healthy mind (Νοῦς ὑγιὴς ἐν σώματι ὑγιεῖ, Thales; in Latin *mens sana in corpore sano*), and with Athene (Pausanias).

It is significant that Pandora's vase was sent to the human race at Zeus's command just after Prometheus's theft. Only then does differentiation of the Nosoi as factors external to the self become possible. Only Elpis, hope, is, by Zeus's will, so to speak, 'constitutive', in that she remained 'in the unbreakable house, under the lip of the jar, and did not fly away' (Hesiod). Hesiod also reports that Zeus deprived the Nosoi of the power of speech, so that diseases come in silence; their forewarning will be a slight feeling of unwellness, a vague presentiment to which one attaches little importance, only to regret it later when the full-blown disease emerges. With the dif-ferentiating and objectifying of disease, the *morbus* becomes the objective evil, something to be eradicated, contrary to life and the contrary of life. *Salus* will henceforth be defined as an absence of illness and freedom from suffering, to be defended by every possible means known to current science; such a univocal heroic mission becomes the founding principle of medicine. With the Romans, the affirmation of a health-conscious lifestyle becomes prevalent, as is shown by the widespread occurrence of mottoes like *salus est vita* (health is life).

Some of these concepts would later be abandoned, while others might be highlighted more strongly, in accordance with the prevailing mood of the times. Today's obsession with cosmetic surgery and the unnatural excesses of plastic surgery might represent degenerations of Aegle, while forgetting Telesphorus might be associated with inability to complete a course of treatment, as a narrative restitution of the relationship of reciprocal dependence, which accords the patient recognition of his increased autonomy and gives the doctor back his simple humanity. So Telesphorus might also represent the pure, humble spirit of service of the medical tradition.[48]

The Hippocratic oath (*Corpus Hippocraticum*, 400 BC) specifically takes Apollo, Asclepius, Hygieia and Panacea as its witnesses. It begins as follows:

> I swear by Apollo Physician and Asclepius and Hygieia and Panaceia and all the gods and goddesses, making them my witnesses, that I will fulfil according to my ability and judgement this oath and this covenant: To hold him who has taught me this art as equal to my parents and to live my life in partnership with him, and if he is in need of money to give him a share of mine, and to regard his offspring as equal to my brothers in male lineage and to teach them this art – if they desire to learn it – without fee and covenant; to give a share of precepts and oral instruction and all the other learning to my sons and to the sons of him who has instructed me and to pupils who have signed the covenant and have taken an oath according to the medical law, but to no one else. I will apply dietetic measures for the benefit of the sick according to my ability and judgement; I will keep them from harm and injustice.[49]

For Hippocrates, the most important figures are Hygieia – the future Salus – and Panacea, the universality of healing of illness.

By contrast, the modern versions of the Oath, with their normative schematism, have a very impersonal style. Here are the opening sentences of the most recent version issued by the Central Committee of the National Federation of the Italian Order of Surgeons and Dental Surgeons (2014):

> Conscious of the importance and solemnity of the act that I am performing and of the commitment I am making, I swear: – to practise medicine with autonomy of judgement and responsibility of behaviour, opposing any undue conditioning that might limit the freedom and independence of the profession; – to pursue the defence of life, the protection of physical and psychic health, the treatment of pain and the relief of suffering, always respecting the dignity and freedom of the person to whom I will dedicate every professional action with constant scientific, cultural and social commitment.[50]

This foregoing discussion shows that, by direct analogy or intuitive feeling, Asclepius's offspring point quite clearly towards today's specializations. Not only does medicine become more and more a science, and less and less an art, but within it the qualities of health and illness, old age and youth, equilibrium and disability, move further and further apart. Disease, or *morbus*, the instinctual, unconscious nature originally associated with the chimerical figure of Chiron, is projected outwards and combated; and in the process, every effort to define, pursue and eradicate it is justified. At the same time, medicine loses its polar opposites; it only wants Apollo, and forgets about Dionysus. It prefers to associate with the classicism of art, which sees ancient Greece as a world made up entirely of Apollonian beauties, with the attributes of symmetry, order and harmony. It sweeps away the ugliness of Dionysus and Silenus with a brusque surgical gesture, breaking the link with their 'naked life', zoe and its deformities.[51] Doctors abandon the chimerical nature of Chiron with Prometheus and Hercules, putting all their trust in a formidable *techne* allied with an iron will. They forget the dark fire of Asclepius's maternal ancestry, which will always lie hidden in his heart, implying forgetfulness of Dionysus and, together with him, of the 'great' Pan.

The contradictory riches of the ancient world are presented to the modern world in a new form by Goethe's Dr Faust, when the discovery of the kingdom of the Mothers, a specifically feminine quality of the unknowable world of primordial forms, reveals the great vision of Walpurgis Night.[52] Plutarch had written, in his treatise *The Twilight of the Oracles*, of a 'field of truth' containing the bases (*logoi*), the forms and original images of all that has existed in the past and will exist in the future. Goethe sees the Mothers as the guardians of the unchanging, eternal essences from which particular existences derive. The great poet of the transition from the Enlightenment to Romanticism sees the encounter with the feminine as a chance of salvation for Faust/Mephistopheles. Walpurgis Night brings a meeting, in a wonderful tangle of visions, between the symbolic universe of the Nordic world and the world of Greek mythology, which is still alive, though dulled and distorted by classicism. The story of earthly love for Gretchen, its destruction by the (dogmatic) spirit of the times and its visionary transfiguration into love for Helen recall Dionysus's affinity with the feminine (the god was surrounded by feminine attention from childhood onwards), reaffirming the spiritual need for his qualities in our nascent era. Curiously enough, it is Chiron himself who shows Faust the road that leads to Helen.

A final example of the evolution of the myth and its terminology is Goethe's Homunculus. Having been fashioned by human hands, he is quite different on the symbolic level from the human being made out of clay by the hands of Prometheus. He stands midway between nostalgia for the first human beings and the coming of artificial human beings. This rational and mythical creature, the Ironic one, the unborn son of Faust's knowledge, introduces Mephistopheles to the Greek mythological universe, and thereby introduces the Devil of monotheism to his Greek precursors. Homunculus explains:

> From place to place I flit and hover
> And, in the best sense, I would fain exist,
> And most impatient am, my glass to shatter.[53]

Thales says of him to Proteus:

> He asks thy counsel, he desires to 'be'.
> He is, as I myself have heard him say,
> (The thing's a marvel!) only born half-way.
> He has no lack of qualities ideal,
> But far too much of palpable and real.
> Till now the glass alone has given him weight,
> And he would fain be soon incorporated.[54]

Homunculus smashes his crystal ball against the shell which once belonged to Venus and now belongs to Galatea, the marine Aphrodite, the origin of life. It is like a visionary, pagan foretaste of the attitude of humankind today: a progressive immersion of knowledge in matter, human thought descending and becoming incarnate in matter. But it is also a pagan antithesis of Faust's salvation; if there is perhaps also an intuition of the insufficiency of technology as a way of saving humankind, and ultimately of its fallibility, this is ignored in the face of the knowledge of pain and death.

With this heroic attitude, technological human beings agree to give up their ancient freedom for the sake of realizing the superhuman potential inherent in technology. Indeed, the loss of that freedom even becomes desirable to them, by voluntary restriction to a mode of knowledge which renounces the risks and uncertainties of imaginary realizations to take refuge in the concrete world of technological matter, where they acquire another form of freedom, but also a great illusion. They arrive not so much at a condition which realizes their own freedom, but at eternal movement longing for freedom from the constraints of the world and for a widening of the boundaries of knowledge.

The wounded healer: the present-day relevance of the myth of Asclepius

> Angels are the powers hidden in the human faculties and organs.
> —Ibn Arabi[55]

At first sight, the symbol of the wounded healer might seem to indicate the empathetic ability to intensify and transform the quality of vision through an intimate feeling and intuition linked to the art of healing. Wounding, in the sense of receiving or inflicting a wound, is indispensable to the process of healing: doctors, in their practice, live in that twilight zone between life and death, recovery and decline. The progress of the treatment is always on the crest of the hill, and may result in unexpected deterioration or even death. The thread of this tension is thin and taut, like that of the surgeon who carries out a delicate operation on which the patient's life depends.

According to Kerényi, Asclepius knows human suffering and is deeply moved by it. The poisoned arrow of suffering and its close link with the mystery of death and the dark side of nature is exactly what lights in his heart and in his eyes a tragic spark, which is linked to an intuitive knowledge of how it is possible to re-emerge from the abyss enriched.[56]

In the art of medicine, both Asclepius, because of the nature of his birth and death, and Chiron, who was struck down by Hercules, and also Machaon, who was mortally wounded in battle, become symbols of the wounded healer. The vital thread of empathy and inexplicable affinities that connects the patient's heart to that of the doctor becomes authentic knowledge of suffering and its treatment. Over the centuries the image of the 'wounded healer' has handed down the traditional function of healing in a higher sense, which includes this intimacy and compassion.

However, as Hillman points out,

> The 'wounded healer' does not mean merely that a person has been hurt and can empathize, which is too obvious and never enough to heal. Nor does it mean that a person can heal because he or she has been through an identical process, for this would not help us unless the process had utterly altered consciousness. Let us remember that the 'wounded healer' is not a human person, but a *personification* presenting a kind of consciousness. This kind of consciousness refers to mutilations and afflictions of the body organs that release the sparks of consciousness in those organs, resulting in an organ or body consciousness. Healing comes then not because one is a whole, integrated, and all together, but from a consciousness breaking through dismemberment.[57]

It is always a sensitively inferior, dissociated, decentralized, and therefore tenuous consciousness. 'When disintegration anxiety is no longer paramount, the compensatory emphasis upon ideals of wholeness, order, and union can fade into the thin spiritualized air that is its *jinn*'.[58] It allows the sensuousness of the discovery of body complexes, which join together the psyche and the libidinal body. 'A wound may be a mouth that speaks spirit, but the spirit is in the flesh'.[59] For what needs to be 'healed' is not just the wound, the disease in a concrete sense, but also a condition of consciousness which is brutally confronted with the stark fact of its own limits. The existential condition of affliction as a way of living in the world is announced through attention to the bodily organ; through every symptom, consciousness is informed of its vulnerability, but also of its links with something that transcends it. This leads to the development of a somatic consciousness, a complementary faculty which, originating in the body, expresses itself as a new mode of consciousness, and invites the ego to pay attention to it, to transform the fear of it starting from its somatic base, heeding the voice coming from the body's habitually silent presence. It is an opportunity: knowing the limit, we can understand its value.

This consciousness of the diseased organ is Dionysus Zagreus, the mutilated Dionysus of classical tragedy, and it is the central element in the archetype of the wounded healer; it indicates the coexistence, alongside the concrete process of treatment, of a second level, consisting of perception and imagination, but especially of containment of tension, and openness to the self, which integrates the sense of limit and mortality. It reveals itself, starting from the suffering of the organ, and requires an initiation into the constant duplicity of individuality, into the asymmetrical dual structure of individual consciousness. 'The experience of the Dyonisian [sic] body is also a death of our own habitual physical frame. Woundedness is initiatory to meeting Dyonisus. It starts us into the subtle body.'[60] Telesphorus and, as Hillman imagines, the mystery rites of the Kabirs in Samothrace, were perhaps a symbolic testimony of it.[61] The aspiration to transcendence and the corporeal signifier on the one hand, and the spiritual quest and signified of the illness on the other, seek each other out and cluster together; recognizing them, encouraging the encounter, is possible. It is not an abstract or conceptual search, but an intuitive, often non-verbal faculty, which leaves a trace. An asymmetry of consciousness, which, if recognized, is both medicine/antidote and poison at the same time.

Experiencing this tension is distinct from the one-sidedness of the unitary concept of the personality, which is the basis of our approach to the patient. Rather than adhering to the dogma of psycho-physical integrity which supports the urgency of the *restitutio ad integrum* and pursues that as its sole task, we could keep our eyes watchful and our ears constantly listening to this ontological signification in the heart of the individual. The symptom conveys a symbolic meaning which 'heals', when it comes to express itself at moments of localized consciousness, which open to the transcendence of the self. This is a dual narrative of a dual path, in which the somatic consciousness of the wound takes shape through the 'inferior function', sees its constant presence behind the scenes, does not ignore it, indeed pursues it, accepts its pace and its needs, and goes on to create and recreate a new balancing point of the somatopsychic tension. The time of waiting, of *incubatio*, is superimposed on technological time, until the momentary exchange between the two levels qualitatively transforms awareness, determining a new attitude.

The dissociative tendency is accepted, within certain limits, because consciousness is 'no longer' situated in the centre. The repeated experience of the encounter with the physicality of the complexes,[62] through the symptom and convalescence, changes the consciousness of one's vulnerability, of one's individual history: the symptom becomes less alarming and the wound may become a scar. The meeting with one's own limit emphasizes the vital thread of one's biography; it experiences 'the inevitability of being wounded in the world', but it makes us free to perceive the emotional value of the dual nature, concrete and imaginal, of life. The concept of healing is replaced by that of *individuation*, the body's opposition to one-sided will and unity is included in it. The individual frame and limitation is accepted by comprehending what transcends it, and opens us to the relation with the infinite.

This approach is different from that of the pure objective hero, immersed in the problem of emancipation from the material and feminine world. The physician who finds himself engaged in the process of treatment needs to reify the patient in the fulfilment of the technological gesture; the surgeon who has to carry out a long and complex operation may need to draw on heroic energies. There is no intention here to deny the at least momentary necessity of adopting a heroic position. The point is that one may realize being able to change this position, and also to listen to the patient, to open up to that second level, making an authentic intersubjective relationship possible. The technological moment and a heroic position are necessary, but can progress from being circumscribed within a univocal, paradigmatic choice. If we transcend the logic of the either-or, we finally open the door to the feminine which nourishes, sustains, mitigates and protects, in its maternal sense, or which is desired, imagined and vitalizing, in its sense of anima. It becomes an ally, as Nausicaa was to Ulysses or as Asclepius's daughters – and the natural forces that they represent – are to each patient every day. This integration helps to open the ego to a dimension that relativizes the symptom, accepts its autonomy, the asymmetric ontological inequality in 'the disharmonies we feel as longings'.[63]

The development of this faculty of operating on two levels may concern both the doctor and the patient. The patient will be helped by the doctor, who is able to sense and respect these moments of corporeal consciousness. The doctor, for his part, can help put those moments into words and, on the basis of the patient's response, develop a dialogue on a different level, a language that relativizes the illness without denying it, creating an ironic distance, a buffer zone embracing both acceptance and imagination. Irony is cathartically linked to double significance, and can start the paradigmatic shift.

In reality, this kind of encounter occurs constantly, thanks to the natural abilities of doctors and patients, without any specific or abstract preparation. What perhaps is lacking is constancy in the quest for this level – attention to it on a collective level which can help to guide choices or modify them as it goes (since the 'health authority' is not organized around this level, but around the level of action, there is bound to be a spontaneous compensation). For when it is a question of choosing, the schema that always prevails is that of diagnosis, which necessarily implies a prognosis and determines a therapeutic automatism, because it is entrusted to the powerful collective hands of the techno-capitalist apparatus.

An imagination that frees and relativizes the relationship between doctor and patient will not take shape as long as we remain one-sidedly anchored to the heroic paradigm of medicine and the concretistic approach.

According to Medicare data for 2001, about 5 per cent of all patients account for 43 per cent of overall expenditure.[64] These are the chronically ill, who are constantly going in and out of hospital because of repeated 'pathological events'; many become dependent on hospitals and spend most of their time there. Not rarely, among these patients, does one come across an intelligent detachment, veiled with irony and relativism, with regard to the technicism of the doctors and the mechanicalness of the administrators. Perhaps we should encourage such patients to help create the models, to rewrite and rephrase a new narrative, whose manifold contributions might surprise us.

The kind of narrative that is typically underlined in our times is a heroic or 'warlike' one, and is accompanied by the myth of its 'real' empirical efficacy. The 'will to live' most often becomes one-sided, leading to over-treatment and overzealousness, as was mentioned earlier. But it is the doctors' task to accept their own vulnerability and fallibility in the first place. As Güggenbuhl-Craig states in his study of power and the helping professions, denying that vulnerability and fallibility may induce doctors to project their own denial on to patients, rather than activating the doctor that exists inside every patient and the patients' capacity for self-treatment.[65] The organizational system, too, must focus on this question of vulnerability, both of the individual doctor and of the organization, which comprises a multiplicity of human beings.

Otherwise, as often happens, doctors will find themselves alone and torn by a conflict between their duty to themselves, in a system which tends not to acknowledge their fallibility, and their duty of treatment, dominated by a concern with efficiency and results.

In this case, the 'Asclepius complex' is constellated in the consuming dualism of burn-out, the slow but relentless fire of the dehumanization of work. Or there may be an inability to give up the idea of saving the patient (and therefore redeeming oneself), whatever the situation, even at the cost of therapeutic excess. Or there may be an obsession with the logic of numbers, a univocal modality which makes the patient a passive receptacle of the doctor's task. In all such cases, there is a forced meeting of the two poles of the therapeutic relationship, through a short-circuit of power, where the doctor is 'only' a doctor, the patient 'only' a patient. In the doctor the patient will not be activated: he or she will not be able to feel with, or for, the patient; and in the patient the doctor will not be activated to restore freedom and integrity.

In the most serious form of the complex, the doctor's main defence is cynicism. He or she performs pointless operations, or ones of doubtful efficacy, lapsing into a form of omnipotence. In such cases, immorality precedes omnipotence, driven by market pressure and hidden by an iron curtain behind the altar of science. These attitudes may account for part of the 'systemic waste', which does not lead to better health and perhaps still eludes our present criteria of evaluation.

This blood flows because of the sacrifice of Chiron and the loss of the sense of limit, which was well known to the tension of his nature. The outcome of mortality and sickness – that is, the 'hard end-points' of medical studies on effectiveness, might be blurred and softened, at least in the case of elderly patients, by a dimension which attaches central importance to quality of life and dignity, in the face of the possibility of death. For insisting on life-saving procedures may emphasize death, beyond bringing it to the instant time of operational risk – accepts a few possible deaths today in exchange for many lengthened diseases tomorrow. It condemns patients without warning – and often with a limited objective – and then insists on redeeming them, thereby appropriating their illusory freedom. In contrast, the tragic sparkle of Asclepius's vision, which does not surrender to the market, and helps patients to contain their fear, is something that all doctors can still achieve and feel in their hearts.

Notes

1 Zoja 2010, pp. 3–12 (Italian edition only).
2 Jaspers 1949, p. 24:

> *Four times* man seems, as it were, to have started out *from a new basis.* First from prehistory, from the Promethean age that is scarcely accessible to us (genesis of speech, of tools and of the use of fire), through which he

first became man. Secondly, from the establishment of the ancient civilisations. Thirdly, from the Axial Period through which, spiritually, he unfolded his full human potentialities. Fourthly, from the scientific-technological age, whose remoulding effects we are experiencing in ourselves.

3 Kerényi 1948.
4 Ibidem.
5 Ibidem.
6 Kerényi 1951, p. 257.
7 Nietzsche 1872, pp. 3–4.
8 Kerényi 1948.
9 Before becoming the emblem of Hermes/Mercury, the caduceus had been associated with Hermes Trismegistus, the legendary progenitor of alchemy in the Hellenistic age, and represented the synthesis of universal knowledge, religion, medicine, ethics, philosophy, the sciences and mathematics. The winged rod around which two serpents, one male and one female, poison and antidote, twined – with cyclical and symmetrically opposite coils, indicating the bidirectionality of time that is resolved in the present time of the wand – is the first *symbolon*, the herald of the messenger of the Gods and mediator in disputes, Mercury. It contains within it the polarity that unites the chthonian principle and the solar one. The wings may indicate the transforming power of the symbol itself, in the metaphorical space of the containment of the metaphysical tension of the opposites. So the form of the caduceus contrasts with the spirit of concretism, substituting the containment of tension for its 'unleashing'. In its quality as a mediator in disputes and because of Mercury's unscrupulousness and volatility, the caduceus justifiably became a symbol of trade and exchange. Asclepius's rod is different. Its single serpent may indicate the hidden treasure, the possibility of the enrichment of the personality that derives from the conscious integration of the inferior function, which has remained isolated, split. On the material level, it may represent the emergence of medicine from the secrets of matter, as knowledge of the therapeutic properties of medicinal herbs. As was mentioned earlier, Asclepius and his family are on friendly terms with the serpent, as is shown in numerous sculptures of the god and his daughter Hygieia carrying a serpent in their arms. This may therefore also indicate the art of medicine's rootedness in the feminine principle (Aristotelian substance or the *prima materia* of alchemy), which tends towards the revitalization of the spirit – towards the *homo totus*, which is the larger personality into which the patient's enriched awareness can evolve. This is the tendency of the ego that suffers and, in the case of illness, is oppressed by superimposed levels of circumstances and tensions arranged around a centre, the self, connected to the hand of fate or of *individuation*, in other words to the hand of the god who holds the top of the wand. In 1902 Mercury's caduceus was adopted as the symbol of the Medical Department of the United States Army. It was also used for a short time by the American Medical Association, though they later abandoned it in favour of Asclepius's rod. But the caduceus emblem still remains on the uniforms of medical officers of the American army and there has been widespread replication of this error all over the nation, which has made it the commonest medical symbol in North America. This confusion between the two symbols seems to be facilitated by the typically modern tendency to confuse symbols with signs – to the predominance, that is, of literal interpretation.
10 See Jung 1911–12, *Symbols of Transformation*, in 'The Dual Mother', p. 374.
11 Ibidem, p. 374.
12 Ibidem, p. 374.

13 Ibidem, p. 354:

> For the hero, fear is a challenge and a task, because only boldness can deliver from fear. And if the risk is not taken, the meaning of life is somehow violated, and the whole future is condemned to hopeless staleness, to a drab grey lit only by will-o'-the-wisps.

14 Ibidem, p. 356.
15 On repression, see Laplanche and Pontalis 1973, pp. 392–396.
16 Kerényi 1948.
17 Nietzsche 1872, p. 116.
18 Plato, *Phaedo*, p. 72.
19 Hillman 1965, p. 157.
20 Nietzsche 1872, p. 78.
21 Ibidem, p. 76.
22 Ibidem, p. 79.
23 Jaspers 1949, p. 2:

> What is new about this age, in all three areas of the world, is that man becomes conscious of Being as a whole, of himself and his limitations. He experiences the terror of the world and his own powerlessness. He asks radical questions. Face to face with the void he strives for liberation and redemption. By consciously recognizing his limits he sets himself the highest goals. He experiences absoluteness in the depths of selfhood and in the lucidity of transcendence. All this took place in reflection. Consciousness became once more conscious of itself, thinking became its own object. Spiritual conflicts arose, accompanied by attempts to convince others through the communication of thoughts, reasons and experiences. The most contradictory possibilities were essayed. Discussion, the formation of parties and the division of the spiritual realm into opposites which nonetheless remained related to one another, created unrest and movement to the very brink of spiritual chaos. In this age were born the fundamental categories within which we still think today, and the beginnings of the world religions, by which human beings still live, were created. The step into universality was taken in every sense. As a result of this process, hitherto unconsciously accepted ideas, customs and conditions were subjected to examination, questioned and liquidated. Everything was swept into the vortex. In so far as the traditional substance still possessed vitality and reality, its manifestations were clarified and thereby transmuted.

24 Natoli 1986, pp. 53–55. For Nietzsche, Prometheus's hubris – his original, active sin – lies in his attempt to pass beyond the bounds of individuation (here understood as a *principium individuationis*, presided over everywhere by Apollo), for 'With the heroic effort made by the individual for universality, in his attempt to [. . .] become the *one* universal being, he experiences in himself the primordial contradiction concealed in the essence of things, i.e., he trespasses and suffers.' For again the fundamental conflict of opposites manifests itself to him 'as a medley of different worlds, for instance, a Divine and a human world, each of which is in the right individually, but as a separate existence alongside of another has to suffer for its individuation' (Nietzsche 1872, p. 79).
25 Nietzsche 1872, p. 34.
26 Zoja 2010, p. 7.
27 Ibidem, pp. 8, 9 (quoted from Pindar, Pythian 2, 42), 11, and 11–12.
28 Hillman 1972, chapter 9, pp. xliv–lvi.

29 Ibidem, p. xlvi.
30 Ibidem, p. lii.
31 Jung 1960, p. 117.
32 Hillman 1981, p. 14:

> And so the task is less to take back these kinds of projections (who takes them back and where are they put?) but more to leap after the projectile reclaiming it as imagination, thereby recognizing that *himma* demands that images always be experienced as sensuous independent bodies.

33 Hillman 1972, p. xxii.
34 Neumann 1956, pp. 28–29, 97.
35 Hillman 1972, p. xxiii.
36 Hillman 1972, p. xxiii.
37 Jaspers 1951, p. 203.
38 Neumann 1949, pp. 286–287:

> Centroversion is the innate tendency of a whole to create unity within its parts and to synthesize their differences in unified systems. [. . .] At a later stage centroversion manifests itself as a directive center, with the ego as the center of consciousness and the self as the psychic center.

39 Jung 1959, p. 227.
40 A Hegelian attitude which underlies historicism and the ideas of progress and evolution. It had a profound influence on the structure of Jung's vision and distorted his perception of the Other as 'primitive' or 'archaic', giving his thought a colonial or ethnocentric tinge. This prejudice can be traced back to founders of the Enlightenment like Voltaire and Kant, who were followed by many later western thinkers such as Fichte and Hegel. Its epitome was the justification of black slavery through the equation of the 'Negro' with a wild, animal-like, non-human or quasi-human being. This is the basis of the reification of 'coloured' humanity, a clearly non-universal definition of what is human. A projection of the split that was mentioned above, it had played a part in the creation of liberal capitalism from the sixteenth century onwards. See Mbembe 2001.
41 Derrida 1968, pp. 128–134.
42 Ibidem, p. 91. Derrida defines hypomnesis as 're-memoration, recollection, consignation'.
43 Ibidem, p. 133. This may be expanded into the idea of deconstruction as a continuous process, one that is necessary if one wishes to embrace a more inclusive concept of history.
44 Zoja 1985, chapter 5: 'Death and Rebirth, and the Death of Rebirth', p. 57.
45 Neumann 1949, p. 321:

> Fragmentation occurs in the sense that, for consciousness, the primordial archetype breaks down into a sizable group of related archetypes and symbols. Or rather, this group may be thought of as the periphery enclosing an unknown and intangible center. The split-off archetypes and symbols are now easier to grasp and assimilate, so that they no longer overpower ego consciousness.

46 Jung 1921, p. 456.

> PARTICIPATION MYSTIQUE is a term derived from Lévy-Bruhl. It denotes a peculiar kind of psychological connection with objects, and consists in the fact that the subject cannot clearly distinguish himself from the object but is bound to it by a direct relationship which amounts to partial identity.

47 *Orphic Hymn* 67 to Hygieia.
48 Telesphorus is also mentioned in connection with the figure of the Kabeiroi, one of the most ancient chthonic deities, associated with the earth, whose cult was widespread from Thebes to Lemnos and Samothrace. These deities fascinated some of the greatest thinkers of German Idealism, from Goethe to Creuzer, and from Schiller to Jung. They were the centre of mystery rites of male initiation, in Samothrace. These 'little people', of whom there were an indeterminate number, are transformed in Goethe's *Faust* into comic figures of elves, pygmies, ants or crabs. According to Diodorus Siculus they are the fingers of the Great Mother of Mount Ida, in Phrygia (*Idaioi daktyloi*). Patrons of secret arts, possessors of a 'ridiculous wisdom', they represent for Jung a symbol of psychic energy, in his conception of the libido (Jung 1911–12, pp. 126–129). Jung carved a statue of Telesphorus in the garden of his country house at Bollingen. In the chapter on the concept of quaternity in *Psychology and Religion* (Jung 1938, p. 164) they are the fourth function or inferior function. In *Memories, Dreams, Reflections* (Jung 1961, p. 227) he describes how he carved the statue in the garden of the Tower of Bollingen:

> I began to see on the front face, in the natural structure of the stone, a small circle, a sort of eye, which looked at me. I chiseled it into the stone, and in the center made a tiny homunculus. This corresponds to the 'little doll' (*pupilla*) yourself which you see in the pupil of another's eye; a kind of Kabir, or the Telesphoros of Asklepios. Ancient statues show him wearing a hooded cloak and carrying a lantern. At the same time he is a pointer of the way.

As Goethe puts it in *Faust*: 'These incomparable, unchainable, Are always further yearning, / With desire and hunger burning / For the unattainable!' (Goethe 1808 and 1832, p. 151; Part II, lines 8202–8205, in the German text). And Jung goes on:

> Myths which day has forgotten continue to be told by night, and powerful figures which consciousness has reduced to banality and ridiculous triviality are recognized again by poets and prophetically revived; therefore they can also be recognized 'in changed form' by the thoughtful person. The great ones of the past have not died, as we think; they have merely changed their names.

'Small and slight, but great in might, the veiled Kabir enters a new house' (Jung 1961, p. 282). The association with the Kabir (whose Semitic etymological origin, 'the great', is significantly paradoxical) makes Telesphorus the most mysterious of Asclepius's children. Forgetting Telesphorus might be linked to the spread and maintenance of the consumeristic shadow of medicine, since without it, as was mentioned earlier, the patient will not regain his capacity for self-healing and re-entering the flow of life. The unidirectionality in the therapeutic relationship, that of the patient who presents himself as an object, will be made artificially eternal; it will never be able to reach an end.
49 Amnesty International 2009, p. 3.
50 FNOMCeO 2014 website, downloadable document in Italian.
51 This unconscious tone is projected into racism by the unconscious perception of the other, the different person and the migrant as ugly, stupid and dangerous.
52 Goethe 1808 and 1832, Part II, pp. 103–227.
53 Goethe 1808 and 1832, p. 136 (Part II, lines 7830–7833, in the German text).
54 Ibidem, p. 153 (Part II, lines 8246–8252, in the German text).
55 Muḥyiddin Ibn Arabi is a thirteenth-century Sufi mystic, and a saint of Islam.
56 Kerényi 1948, p. 69:

> It is neither a religious nor a philosophical knowledge; indeed it cannot be set down as any sort of departmentalized knowledge, but it is rather a familiarity

which can never be acquired, with sickness and the process of recovery. It is a spark of intuitive knowledge about the possibilities of rising from the depths, a spark which by observation, practice and training, can be fanned into a high art and science, into a true art of healing. The religion of the Koan physicians was directed toward this spark and its sun-like efflorescence.

57 Hillman 2005, p. 234.
58 Ibidem, p. 234.
59 Ibidem, p. 235.
60 Ibidem, p. 235.
61 Ibidem, pp. 185–191.
62 On the complex, see Laplanche and Pontalis 1973, pp. 72–74.
63 Hillman 2005, p. 190. The mighty ones, the Kabirs of Samothrace, are an archetypal representation of this; their arrival represents the recognition of the metaphorical man, who, 'unlike literal man fixed in his certainties, is always at sea, always en route between, always in two places at once.'
64 Fineberg 2012.
65 Guggenbühl-Craig 1971, pp. 83–87.

Bibliography

Amnesty International (2009), *Codes of Ethics and Declarations Relevant to the Health Professions: An Amnesty International Compilation of Selected Ethics and Human Rights Texts and Other International Standards*, London: Amnesty International Ltd., Fifth Edition, 2011 [c. 2009].

Derrida, Jacques (1968), *'Plato's Pharmacy'*, in *Dissemination*, translated with an introduction and additional notes by Barbara Johnson, London: The Athlone Press, 1993. The translation was first published by The University of Chicago Press, 1981.

Eliot, Thomas Stearns (1943), 'East Coker', in *Four Quartets*, London: Faber and Faber Limited, 1983.

Fineberg, Harvey V. (2012), 'A Successful and Sustainable Health System: How to Get There from Here', *New England Journal of Medicine*, 366 (2012), pp. 1020–1027.

FNOMCeO (Federazione Nazionale degli Ordini dei Medici Chirurghi e Odontoiatri: National Federation of the Italian Order of Surgeons and Dental Surgeons) (2014), *Giuramento professionale*. https://portale.fnomceo.it/fnomceo/Giuramento+professionale. html?t=a&id=145135 Accessed 30th October 2017.

Goethe, Johann Wolfgang von (1808 and 1832), *Faust: Eine Tragödie. Faust: A Tragedy*, Parts I & II, translated by Bayard Taylor, Boston & New York: Houghton Mifflin Co., 1870.

Guggenbühl-Craig, Adolf (1971), *Macht als Gefahr beim Helfer. Power in the Helping Professions*, translated by Myron Gubitz, Putnam, CT: Spring Publications, 2009.

Hillman, James (1965), *Suicide and the Soul*, Woodstock, CT: Spring Publications, 1997.

Hillman, James (1972), 'An Essay on Pan', in *Pan and the Nightmare*, (the only English Translation – from the German by A.V. O'Brien, M.D. – of *Ephialtes: A Pathological-Mythological Treatise on Nightmare in Classical Antiquity*, by Wilhelm Heinrich Roscher, 1900 together with *An Essay on Pan*, serving as Psychological Introduction to Roscher's *Ephialtes*), New York: Spring Publications, 1972.

Hillman, James (1981), *The Thought of the Heart and the Soul of the World*, Woodstock, CT: Spring Publications, 1997.

Hillman, James (2005), *Senex & Puer*, Uniform Edition of the Writings of James Hillman, Volume 3, Connecticut: Spring Publications, 2005.

Jaspers, Karl (1949), *Vom Ursprung und Ziel der Geschichte. The Origin and Goal of History*, translated by Michael Bullock, New Haven & London: Yale University Press, 1953.

Jaspers, Karl (1951), *Strindberg und van Gogh: Versuch einer Pathographischen Analyse. Strindberg and Van Gogh: An Attempt at a Pathographic Analysis with Reference to Parallel Cases of Swedenborg and Hölderlin*, translated by Oskar Grunow and David Woloshin, Tucson, AZ: University of Arizona Press, 1977.

Jung, Carl Gustav (1911–12), *Symbole der Wandlung: Analyse des Vorspiels zu einer Schizophrenie. Symbols of Transformation: An Analysis of the Prelude to a Case of Schizophrenia*, Bollingen Series XX, Vol. 5 of the Collected Works of C.G. Jung, translated by Richard Francis Carrington Hull, Princeton, NJ: Princeton University Press, 1967.

Jung, Carl Gustav (1921), *Psychologische Typen. Psychological Types*, Bollingen Series XX, Vol. 6 of the Collected Works of C.G. Jung, A revision by Richard Francis Carrington Hull of the translation by Helton Godwin Baynes, Princeton, NJ: Princeton University Press, 1971.

Jung, Carl Gustav (1938), *Zur Psychologie Westlicher und östlicher Religion. Psychology and Religion, West and East*, Bollingen Series XX, Vol. 11 of the Collected Works of C.G. Jung, translated by Richard Francis Carrington Hull, Princeton, NJ: Princeton University Press, 1958.

Jung, Carl Gustav (1959), *Die Archetypen und das Kollektive Unbewußte. The Archetypes and the Collective Unconscious*, Bollingen Series XX, Vol. 9, Part I of the Collected Works of C.G. Jung, translated by Richard Francis Carrington Hull, Princeton, NJ: Princeton University Press, 1969.

Jung, Carl Gustav (1960), *Die Dynamik des Unbewußten. The Structure and Dynamics of the Psyche*, Bollingen Series XX, Vol. 8 of the Collected Works of C.G. Jung, translated by Richard Francis Carrington Hull, in *Psychological Factors in Human Behaviour* (1936), Princeton, NJ: Princeton University Press, 1969.

Jung, Carl Gustav (1961), *Erinnerungen Träume Gedanken. Memories, Dreams, Reflections*, recorded and edited by Aniela Jaffé, translated from the German by Richard and Clara Winston, New York: Vintage Books Edition, A Division of Random House, 1989.

Kerényi, Karol (1948), *Der göttliche Arzt: Studien über Asklepius und seine Kultstätte. Asklepios: Archetypal Image of the Physician's Existence*, Bollingen Series, Vol. LXV.3, New York: Pantheon Books, 1959.

Kerényi, Karl (1951), *Die Mythologie der Griechen. The Gods of the Greeks*, London: Thames & Hudson, 2008.

Laplanche, Jean & Pontalis, Jean-Bertrand (1973), *The Language of Psycho-Analysis*, with an introduction by Daniel Lagache, translated by Donald Nicholson-Smith, London: Hogarth Press, 1973.

Mbembe, Achilles (2001), *Notes Provisoires sur la Postcolonie. On the Postcolony (Studies on the History of Society and Culture)*, translated by A.M. Berrett, Janet Roitman, Murray Last, and Steven Rendall, Berkeley, CA: University of California Press, 2001.

Natoli, Salvatore (1986), *L'Esperienza del Dolore, Le Forme del Patire nella Cultura Occidentale. The Experience of Pain: The Forms of Suffering in Western Culture*, Milan: Feltrinelli, 2008.

Neumann, Erich (1949), *Ursprungsgeschichte des Bewusstseins. The Origins and History of Consciousness*, Bollingen Series XLII, translated by Richard Francis Carrington Hull, Princeton, NJ: Princeton University Press, 1954.

Neumann, Erich (1956), *Amor und Psyche, mit einem Kommentar von Erich Neumann: Ein Beitrag zur seelischen Entwicklung des Weiblichen. Amor and Psyche: The Psychic Development of the Feminine: A Commentary on the Tale by Apuleius*, Bollingen Series LIV, translated from the German by Ralph Manheim, Princeton, NJ: Princeton University Press, 1956.

Nietzsche, Friedrich (1872), *Die Geburt der Tragödie. Oder: Griechenthum und Pessimismus. The Birth of Tragedy, or Hellenism and Pessimism*, translated by William August Haussmann, Auckland, New Zealand: The Floating Press, 2016.

Orpheus, *The Hymns of Orpheus*, translated by Thomas Taylor (1792), Philadelphia: University of Pennsylvania Press, 1999.

Plato, *Phaedo*, translated with notes by David Gallop, Oxford: Oxford University Press, 1975.

Zoja, Luigi (1985), *Nascere Non Basta, Iniziazione e Tossicodipendenza. Drugs, Addiction and Initiation, the Modern Search for Ritual*, translated by Marc E. Romano and Robert Mercurio, 2012, Einsiedlen, Switzerland: Daimon Verlag, 2000.

Zoja, Luigi (2010), *Centauri, Miti e Violenza Maschile*, Bari: Editori Laterza, 2010.

Chapter 2

Alfred Ziegler's archetypal medicine[1]

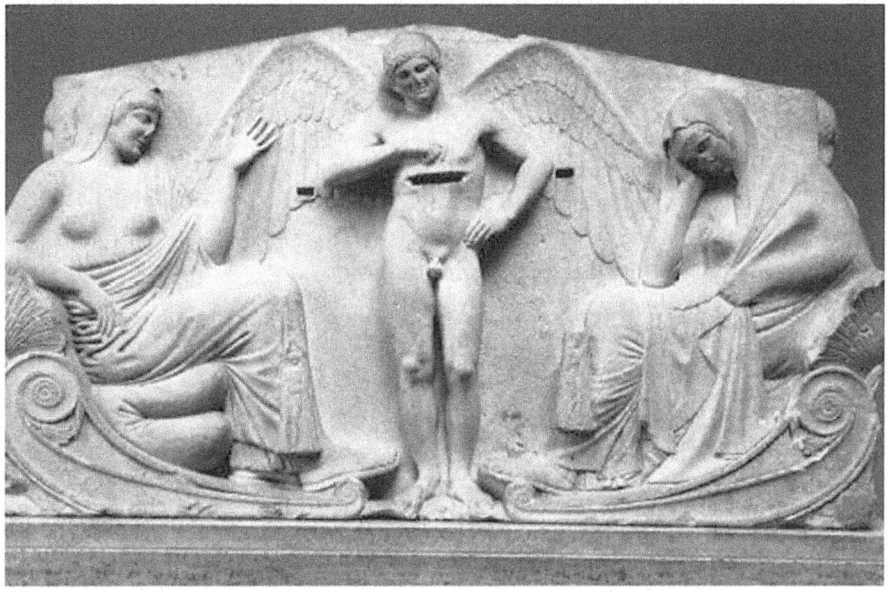

Figure 2.1 Thanatos between Aphrodite and Persephone. Burstein collection/Corbis.
Unknown photographer.

Death and life, love and death, constantly intertwine like polar comple-
ments of a single indefinable phenomenon, which we tend to call simply
life, whereas it is in fact incommunicable tension over the abyss, horror and
sublime, germination and decomposition, constantly and intimately linked
and dissolved. Life's very exuberance expresses a disposition to decay, a programme interwoven into the letters and particles of which life is made up.
In this sense, birth already contains within itself a narrative of a thousand
possible deaths. It is the exuberance and one-sidedness of living which is
constantly expressed and mitigated, and which records in the environment,

under the guise of illness, a certain number of possible 'deaths'. The causal factor is not important; it is gathered in by the soul to the extent that every illness is an opportunity for life to renew itself or perish. The capacity to see physical symptoms from this viewpoint makes them vehicles of meaning in a process which makes the body resemble an alchemical *opus*. The body becomes a subtle body, and each stage is part of a process tending towards individuation, in a dimension that no longer distinguishes subject and object, inside and outside, but merges them in the language of the symbols that comprise or transcend them.

A medicine based on the principle of polarity starts from the conscious experience of the inherent symbolic tension between sickness and health. In it, value is attached to the thanatotropic tendency (from *thanatos*, death, and *tropos*, turning towards) intrinsic to life, which emerges in our culture in various symbolisms linked to personified death. In Goethe's *Faust*, Mephistopheles describes himself as follows:

> Part of that Power, not understood,
> Which always wills the Bad, and always works the Good. [. . .]
> I am the Spirit that Denies!
> And justly so: for all things, from the Void
> Called forth, deserve to be destroyed:
> 'Twere better, then, were naught created.
> Thus, all which you as Sin have rated,
> – aught with Evil blent, –
> That is my proper element.[2]

By denying the shadow[3] and the inferior functions of the personality and persisting in the dominant attitude of good health, in the univocal exuberance of the 'healthy life', in varying degrees and at different times these repressed functions materialize as symptoms. The demons (*daimones*) of illness 'fall into the soma' and the individual will be inhabited, so to speak, by an outside will, which desires its destruction. The soul will communicate with the Devil through the diseases, his mediators. The more the individual persists in a one-sided attachment to health, the greater will be the opposition of a contrasting irrational force, which at a certain point plunges into the soma to undermine dominant values, oppose habits, overturn intentions. So 'archetypal' medicine sides with the demon; it is with him that it communicates, aiming to preserve and refine his presence and understand his language, always remaining close to the body. Since the method adopted is dialogue based on introverted intuition – in contrast to the extroverted thought of empirical medicine – we are presented with seemingly unconnected images of the illness and the symptom, which, as if in an alchemical process, 'extract' or 'sublimate' what is essential in them. Archetypal medicine aims at the symbolic meaning of illness; its tools are communicative language and a love of etymology and amplification, in the context of a process which is careful to avoid any concretistic and causalistic temptation, where the doctor is the communicating vehicle of the cure. The doctor starts from a sensual rooting of language in the body, the verification of which is the actual correspondence, felt by the patient, of images evoked by symptoms and physical perceptions. The rooting of this 'cure of the word' in the body is the foundation of an approach which proceeds by similarities, which arise by chance in the course of a dialogue whose direct object is never the symptom. The main ethical value of this approach to the meaning of illness is lightness, in a constellation of fragments, of intuitions, which go beyond nosology and the bounds of causality. Whereas empirical medicine makes use mainly of thought and sensation, nosological classification and technology, 'archetypal' medicine makes use of intuition, with its discontinuity, and of emotion, which is able to verify the correct value of images and store it up for the future. Its god is the volatile Hermes; his is the Mercurial element, antithetical to the Apollonian. Ziegler points out that the ethic of empirical medicine is based on education, on the memorizing of a large number of rational and empirical facts, where causality and the risk of error are the main determining factors: a deeply serious ethic, where the value of the 'objective fact' is fundamental and invests the doctor with responsibility for the most precise formulations, the most objective processes, the antithesis of vagueness and subjectivity. Archetypal medicine, by contrast, starts from a level where your view becomes blurred, as if you were squinting slightly, to conjure out of the mist a relative view of the illness, a momentary ironic detachment from the symptom, which gives value also to the irrational and emotional side of the human being.

When someone falls ill, the soul, which in analytical psychology is the medium through which the individual can communicate with the unconscious and give expression to the inferior functions, 'falls' into the body, because expression has been denied to the recessive traits for too long, and with varying degrees of intensity. We all have dissonances, deformations, inabilities, shadows, but we also have strange unexpected gifts, which others can see much better than us. When these aspects of the personality have been constantly repressed for too long, they 'fall' into the body. With the arrival of somatization, they orient differently the conscious attitude and the adolescent exuberance of life, bringing with them unexpected, hitherto unknown meanings. Illness forces the conscience to stop and listen to the new voices, which have had no other way of expressing themselves than through the soma.

In this connection, the chorus from Aeschylus's *Agamemnon* is relevant:

> Health [Hygieia], to largeness growing, will not rest
> Safe within limit; yet the verge is pressed
> By neighbour Sickness, one thin wall between:
> Ships in full career and fates alike
> In prosperous weather unawares will strike
> Upon a reef unseen.[4]

Life unfolds everywhere, like a planned programme of continual compensation for all one-sidedness, for every instance of 'over-florid health'. The body absorbs the appropriate pathogenic *noxae* from the environment. Clearly this process is bound to end ultimately in death, but there is no linear progression, no natural and progressive decline; it happens discontinuously; death is constantly being postponed, and old age is seen as an incurable illness (*senectus ipsa est morbus*).[5] Life, however, communicates with death from the beginning, in a common circular dimension made up of continual processes of destruction and regeneration, 'Formation, Transformation, / Eternal minds in eternal recreation.'[6] There can be no joy without suffering, no life without destruction and eternal recreation. The aetiology is only the pretext, as if the 'cause' of an illness were caught in the environment by chance as a result of an innate predisposition to decay. The consciousness is overwhelmed by a process which starts from the body, and reformulates an idea of health for everyone by accepting what, in the illness, is trying to express itself, what completes the individual, indicates their uniqueness, their irreplaceable nature in the face of death. In a sense, health is considered largely unconscious, for not only does it include illness in its experience, but its greatest realization corresponds to the 'gold in the mud' that illness carries with it and expresses.

Illness has an insidious tendency to manifest itself with varying but predetermined degrees of severity. This process is regulated by pre-established laws of materialization. Each of us has a specific modality that regulates our 'decay'. These 'laws' also guide the realization of our well-being, understood as relief at the discovery of the limit that reveals itself to us. This individuative value of illness has its linguistic and symbolic testament in the bodily organs, and can often be related to the etymology of many morbid conditions, which Ziegler analyses in the practical section of his book.[7] According to Ziegler, it is possible to overcome the one-sidedness of the motto 'salus est vita' through language. Dialogue with the patient aims at identifying the essential characteristic of the symptom, starting from etymology and the amplification of symbols; in the symbolic reflection there is a sudden correspondence by analogy, an instantaneous effect which dilutes, alleviates, and transforms the density and weight of the illness. As mentioned earlier, this can only happen when the word is sufficiently impregnated with the physical and material sensations of the illness – that is to say, it presupposes a pre-verbal process of feeling, expression and communication.[8] The skill lies in avoiding both the concretism of empirical science and the abstraction of pure philosophy. Understanding and assimilation is gradual, through the repetition of the experience, in a process of convalescence which can thus lead to a richer dimension in existence and to the possibility of a new attitude in life.

Unlike empirical medicine, archetypal medicine operates in closed systems, where the elements are always arranged according to polarities and never univocally determined; as was mentioned above, its ethic is relativistic and ironic. In it, everything is only half-real, as if the intentions of nature were not particularly serious. In this, archetypal medicine is inspired by Hermes, by his Mercurial spirit, whereby every single thing is connected to every other thing, in such a way that the cosmos remains a closed system. Hermes, as we will see later, has a sense of humour which is not at all characteristic of Apollo. Hermes's smile is archaic, and constantly nourished by every kind of persistence, trick and untruth, so that it is never attenuated.

The constant refusal to demonize illness is, like the acceptance of illness as a relativistic, complementary and not antithetical '*morbus*', in itself therapeutic. The concept of '*salus est vita*', when it is hypostasized and taken for granted, induces mechanical interventionism: there is a risk of confusing therapy with an apotropaic action tinged with cynicism, which accords itself absolute justification in its fight against evil. In contrast to interventionism, prevention – the discipline of Hygieia, or hygiene – endeavours to avoid illness, forbidding all exposure, contamination, excess, unorthodoxy and unhealthy curiosity. It places the emphasis on 'risk factors', 'risky behaviour' and exposure to such behaviour. By contrast, archetypal medicine recognizes and gives dignity of meaning to the 'thanatotropic' tendency of life, its turning towards death. Its task is to re-sublimate the materialization of the symptom, to transform it with the language of introverted intuition.

Experience shows how nature wishes to undermine the impulse towards health with increasingly drastic measures, the more obsessive this impulse becomes. Irony must, therefore, intervene before medicine's self-image causes it to become counterproductive. Instead of becoming an over-serious, dejected recruit to the course of treatment, with the sole aim of defeating the illness, conquering destiny and 'humiliating fate', the individual sees 'the power that always means well but acts badly' and forms an alliance with it, creating a cure based on symbolic language, with the aim of 'redeeming' what has fallen into the body in the form of physical illness. 'A serious condition with many hopes becomes an unserious condition, but without hopes.' This does not, in my opinion, exclude the empirical process of treatment, but it does introduce a new critical spirit to it.

This ironical, and at the same time almost masochistic, position towards illness expresses a tendency towards a mystique of suffering and a loving relationship with illness, like an alchemical process of extracting spirit from matter. This does not happen without a *Todeshochzeit* ('marriage with death'), which evokes the general mythologem of something particularly desirable linked to something terrifying, and therefore 'dying' (like the mutilated Dionysus of the previous chapter). This peculiar conjunction occurs when suffering offers no other choice than that of making an alliance, while still alive, with death: inviting it to dance, listening to the music of the encounter with what has finally found expression in illness. Being irreplaceable in the face of pain is also expressed by this, by the fact that the range of possibilities is shrinking, and there is no other possible life than this dying one; and this opens the way to the perspective of a relationship with the infinite. In this experience, the individual, as a suffering being, will be able to experience a sense of eternity, as if individual life has acquired for the first time an unequivocal and incorruptible uniqueness, a particular limitation and at the same time a particular freedom. In the imminent dissolution of form, the individual feels and intuits an ontological unity with *physis*, as if this recognition conferred an intimate, unassailable security, in the fluctuating insecurity of life. This is where the 'mystic marriage' with death lies, well before the end of life and the possibility of an ecstatic, mystic dimension, where the ravages of time scarcely affect us any longer, where rather than euphoria we feel an inner sense of security and tranquillity. By not neglecting the treatment, the individual who falls ill winks at the dance of death – the *Totentanz* – that is part of life, and thereby wins greater freedom. Anyone who has been through an experience of this kind feels a sense of rebirth which they will be able to recognize for the rest of their life, the mystic equivalent of 'reconvalescence'.

Ziegler cites the following example:

> When an infarct patient's condition improves after he has been released from the sinister *machine infernale* of an intensive care unit, he shows all the signs of having experienced a *Todeshochzeit*. He may resolve no longer to invest so much 'heart' in things once felt to be important – until an unheeded hate literally attacks him. If he adopts the perhaps naïve-seeming attitude of not taking things so seriously anymore, he is headed for a *status quo ante*, albeit one in which a certain reserve has taken its place. Reconvalescence, in other words, is a reconstituting in which we take something previously regarded as unworthy or useless and join with it in a kind of sacramental marriage.[9]

This is a long process, punctuated by relapses into the dominant attitude, but each time it reaches a level closer to consciousness, when it is supported by verbal therapy. The free intervals become longer and longer, the relapses shorter and shorter, and, more importantly, less serious or serious-minded, not characterized by a total sense of aporia and hopelessness. And with each reactive revival of the dominant attitude, that attitude will be eroded more naturally.

By contrast, any individual who remains oppressed by the 'gravity' of the diagnosis, which weighs on them like a judicial sentence, will psychologically enter the 'clinic' (from *klinikos*, 'pertaining to a bed'); they will be forced into a horizontal position, like a patient in a hospital who is continually told to remain in a posture consonant with the beds, and only the medical staff are authorized to adopt the erect, dominant position of people who ought to know and pursue the good and overcome evil. Oppressed by the ticking of chronological time, by the monotonous pace of prescriptions, by the logic of suspicion, by the hope of a precise diagnosis and by the rigour of the 'best' treatment, the 'bed-ridden' patient will count the hours and days that must pass before 'recovery', before that medical decree on which their 'dismissal' will depend. The only refuge will be not to be able 'to cope with necessity in its purest form, which is time; the most shameful temptation is to escape it by unawareness or to submit blindly to it.'[10]

The alchemical tradition of the late Middle Ages was capable of an esoteric smile:[11] it remained hidden in the shadow of the rigid monotheistic orthodoxies and their inquisitions. In detaching itself from this, modern medicine has become more cynical, incapable of relativizing illness, of accepting it with a certain degree of freedom. Incapable of 'reflecting' inside illness as an essential complement of instinctual nature, it wages constant war on diseases, training paladins of health and virtue. If illness is not part of life, death becomes the worst of enemies, each diagnosis a sentence, each treatment a verdict. 'Life expectancy' becomes our sword of Damocles, consuming us in the expectation of a saving event, the triumph of good over evil. Medicine takes on a moralizing tone, and life will be oppressed by the immanence of a relentless evil that comes from outside, contaminating and corroding us. An evil suspended in judgement and in waiting:

> Usually, disease is no longer perceived as a shadowy struggle with an offended god or an insulted demon. Rather, remorse or regret sets in when, after the fact, the correlation between a disease or chronic suffering and our lifestyle – something which might have been avoided – becomes apparent. Moral overtones resonate even today in all pathology: responsibility, guilt, punishment, and atonement. In earlier times, such a moralistic perspective of disease stood in relation to socializing norms

and to an individual's connection to the divine. Human hubris, blasphemy against divine order, sacrilegious swearing and malice toward all that a god had created drew down disease as punishment. The model is not only Christian but generally religious and ubiquitous, a primal image of how man perceives the coming and going of disease.[12]

For Ziegler, reconvalescence finally recalls those images of resurrection of Christian origin, where the risen Christ shows all the signs of his recent suffering. His body still bears the indelible marks of the wounds, which give him a spiritual aura, of passing over, a light which transfigures the materiality of the body into something pneumatic.

There remains a doubt that Ziegler's approach, rather than a medicine, may be primarily a psychology, an application of the 'cure of the word' to psychosomatics or to the processing of the experience of illness. Its principles are so distant from the spirit of the times as to be inaccessible, though not incomprehensible, to many patients. It is the doctor's task to seek openings at this level, but sometimes these openings present themselves spontaneously, without any pressure being brought to bear on patients' sensibility and *forma mentis*, and irrespective of their level of education. Many people, however, are rather suspicious of intuitive or imaginal approaches, but the key to most minds, in my opinion, is gentle humour, an easygoing attitude in harmony with the patient, attentive to their every observation or need, with a disinterested light-heartedness and dedication.

I would like to end with a personal reminiscence that has an illustrative and emblematic value for me. F., an elderly architect, came to my department, invited by a colleague of mine in the national health service, with his wife, a university lecturer. They were an open-minded, curious couple. He was non-religious, polite and good-natured, attentive to formalities, with an old-fashioned manner about him. She was religious and committed, with a decisive, disciplined temperament, always polite, devoted to her work and family. Both were characterized by great moral seriousness. I used to see them every year, for a cardiological check-up, without ever finding anything wrong. The results of the basic tests were within normal limits. In November of the year in question, the wife felt the need, for no obvious reason, to have me examine her husband. She wasn't convinced that he was well, even though he exhibited no particular symptoms. I told her the examination could wait until after Christmas, but she insisted on bringing it forward. During the examination I noticed a cardiac murmur that had not been picked up before; the patient and his wife didn't seem entirely surprised. The echocardiogram produced the diagnosis of a serious insufficiency of the mitral valve, which had emerged in the meantime because of the breaking of a *chorda tendinea*, an acute event which is initially tolerated but requires a complex heart operation to repair a valve. Without the operation the patient risks developing a serious heart condition over the ensuing months, which will entail a drastic reduction in life expectancy. My language was still anchored to the terminology of empirical medicine, on a terrain where the weight of responsibility pointed not only to the necessity of treatment, but also to the imperative of numbers, the probabilities of the 'risk/benefit' relationship of the surgical operation. This generated in the patient and his wife a need to rely on emergency treatment, which was invested in their relationship with me, their 'family doctor'. I decided to accept the commitment on the personal and professional level, and introduced the patient to the surgeon, who accepted the indication and himself explained carefully to the couple the nature of the operation and the possible complications. The post-operation period was difficult, with many episodes of disorientation and fluctuation of consciousness, after the extra-corporeal circulation. The patient was often tempted to give way to depressive tendencies, which had in fact been evident even before the operation. His neuro-vegetative reflexes were impaired, with intense fragility and muscular weakness in his legs. Then his mind gradually became active again and he could recognize people; he was constantly stimulated by his wife and daughter, who stayed at his bedside with utter devotion. He recognized me as his doctor, and for me, seeing him look at me, and accepting his family, too, in this non-verbal space, was an intense and moving experience. At one point, in the despair and anguish of his extreme weakness and his reluctance to do his physiotherapy exercises, F. started to joke with me. He had a collection of old swords at home, and when he saw me, he would tell me about imaginary weapons he kept under his bed in expectation of my arrival; I told him he was right to make sure he had some weapons, because I too was armed – with a stethoscope!

Suddenly he had a relapse; a syncope raised fears of a stroke, but it was a false alarm. He was moved to another hospital to continue his rehabilitation. One day I got a phone call from his wife. She was worried about F.; he seemed feeble and demoralized. I went to pay him a visit and found him pale and weak, though he smiled when I arrived. I was taken aback to see how emaciated his face was: he was so thin you could see the skeleton underneath. He spontaneously took the initiative; still smiling, he began to talk about death; he said he would be only too happy to let it take him – it would be a relief. His wife was visibly distressed at his words. But the results from his latest tests indicated that his prospects of recovery were good, provided he found the strength to do his exercises, and the will to live. I impressed this on him, and invited him to come for a walk with me along the corridor.

It was then that my language started to change. Walking arm in arm along the corridor, we developed a light-hearted, humorous complicity; we completely stopped talking about things directly. We would move from the handrail to the support of a door, his legs barely supporting him; I adjusted my pace to his. At one point, as we walked, we joked about the idea of dancing. We reached the waiting room, at the end of the corridor, where we sat down with his wife, who had joined us in the meantime. F. smiled and said there were six 'walking corpses' in his ward; one of them was only a youngster, a mere sixty years old. 'He walks as fast as a train!' Returning to the subject of death and the dance, I mentioned Ziegler's notion of the dance with death. It was like a *Toten* . . . 'I can't remember the word. Can you?' 'A *Totentanz*!' he exclaimed. He knew the image (later he told me he had listened to Arturo Benedetti Michelangeli's performance of Franz Listz's *Totentanz*, a paraphrase of the 'Dies irae', which took him twenty years to compose).[13] It was a moving moment; he was resigned, but no longer depressed. A long, poignant silence ensued. I told him his wife had no intention of letting him go, and neither did I; she was moved, and wept for the first time. When I said goodbye, F. seemed to have more vitality in his eyes and more determination to react. His wife's messages over the next few days reported a mood that was still fluctuating, but distinctly more motivated; it seemed like a slow process of rebirth, with increasingly short relapses. Here is an example: 'Dear doctor, The work done over the last few days on motivating him and making him aware of his improvement is bearing fruit, especially in his willingness to do things. [. . .] Thank you; you'll be amazed next time you see him. There will be some dips, of course, but the important thing is that we've made a start.' Some time later, after a long course of physiotherapy, F. completely recovered his strength.

When he finally left my specialized treatment he offered me an ancient Syrian sword from his personal collection. This account was read and approved by F. and his wife before publication.

Notes

1 Ziegler 1983, see the chapter on Theory, pp. 7–46.
2 Goethe 1808, pp. 54–55 (Part I, lines 1336–1338 and 1338–1344, in the German text).
3 Jung 1961, pp. 398–399:

> Shadow. The inferior part of the personality; sum of all personal and collective psychic elements which, because of their incompatibility with the chosen conscious attitude, are denied expression in life and therefore coalesce into a relatively autonomous 'splinter personality' with contrary tendencies in the unconscious. The shadow behaves compensatorily to consciousness; hence its effects can be positive as well as negative. In dreams, the shadow figure is always of the same sex as the dreamer.

Jung 1959, pp. 284–285: 'The shadow personifies everything that the subject refuses to acknowledge about himself and yet is always thrusting itself upon him directly or indirectly – for instance, inferior traits of character and other incompatible tendencies.' Jung 1951, p. 266:

> The shadow [is] that hidden, repressed, for the most part inferior and guilt-laden personality whose ultimate ramifications reach back into the realm of our animal ancestors and so comprise the whole historical aspect of the unconscious. [. . .] If it has been believed hitherto that the human shadow was the source of all evil, it can now be ascertained on closer investigation that the unconscious man, that is, his shadow, does not consist only of morally reprehensible tendencies, but also displays a number of good qualities, such as normal instincts, appropriate reactions, realistic insights, creative impulses, etc.

Jung 1967, pp. 265–266: One does not become enlightened by imagining figures of light, but by making the darkness conscious. The latter procedure, however, is disagreeable and therefore not popular.
4 Aeschylus, *Agamemnon*, p. 121 (lines 990–994 in the Greek text).
5 Terence, line 575.
6 Goethe 1808 and 1832, p. 69 (Part II, lines 6287–6288, in the German text).
7 Ziegler 1983, see the section on *Praxis*, pp. 47–155.
8 Ibidem, p 31:

> The extent to which our organs determine our *Weltanschauungen* finds testament in our language. Any dealing with language and its history, with etymology, seems to lead to endosomatic sensations, sensations which then remain as the substance for all later formulations. Where etymology fails to penetrate to those sensations, it leaves the impression that its task is but half completed. If the so called Indo-Germanic language roots, for instance, did not coincide with a physical sensation like *angh*, which surfaces in *angina* pectoris or in the German *Drang*, of *Sturm und Drang*, they would seem suspended, ungrounded, and rootless.

9 Ibidem, p. 36.
10 Weil 1933–1943, p. 146.
11 Already in the High Middle Ages, alchemists engaged in a search for the elixir of youth, distinguishing it from the philosopher's stone, the subject of a different line of enquiry.
12 Ziegler 1983, p. 38.
13 Liszt, Franz – Totentanz, Paraphrase on 'Dies Irae' S.126 1/2, www.youtube.com/watch?v=7roz8yORa3w Accessed 30th October 2017.

Bibliography

Aeschylus, *Agamemnon*, with verse translation, introduction and notes by Walter Headlam, edited by A.C. Pearson, Cambridge: Cambridge University Press, 1910.

Goethe, Johann Wolfgang von (1808 and 1832), *Faust: Eine Tragödie. Faust: A Tragedy*, Parts I & II, translated by Bayard Taylor, Boston & New York: Houghton Mifflin Co., 1870.

Jung, Carl Gustav (1951), *Aion: Beiträge zur Symbolik des Selbst. Aion: Researches into the Phenomenology of the Self*, Bollingen Series XX, Vol. 9, Part II of the Collected Works of C.G. Jung, translated by Richard Francis Carrington Hull, Princeton, NJ: Princeton University Press, 1969.

Jung, Carl Gustav (1959), *Die Archetypen und das Kollektive Unbewußte. The Archetypes and the Collective Unconscious*, Bollingen Series XX, Vol. 9, Part I of the Collected Works of C.G. Jung, translated by Richard Francis Carrington Hull, Princeton, NJ: Princeton University Press, 1969.

Jung, Carl Gustav (1961), *Erinnerungen Träume Gedanken. Memories, Dreams, Reflections*, recorded and edited by Aniela Jaffé, translated from the German by Richard and Clara Winston, 1989 Vintage Books Edition, New York: A Division of Random House, 1989.

Jung, Carl Gustav (1967), *Studien über Alchemistische Vorstellungen. Alchemical Studies*, Bollingen Series XX, Vol. 13 of the Collected Works of C.G. Jung, translated by Richard Francis Carrington Hull, Princeton, NJ: Princeton University Press, 1970.

Weil, Simone (1933–43), *Cahiers, Oeuvres Complètes. First and Last Notebooks*, translated by Richard Rees, Eugene, OR: Wipf and Stock Publishers, 1970.

Ziegler, Alfred J. (1983), *Krankheitsbilder. Elemente einer Archetypischen Medizin. Archetypal Medicine*, translated from the German by Gary V. Hartman, Woodstock, CT: Spring Publications, 2000.

Part II

Medicine and society in our time

Chapter 3

Modern myths in medicine

In the first part of this book, I described the archetypal roots of medicine in western culture, relating them to the evolution of the doctor's consciousness. In this second part, I will examine some tendencies of medicine in its interrelationship with 'modern myths' – that is, with the unconscious conditioning that underlies our present-day behaviour and helps to determine choices in the medical field. I will examine the role of doctors with respect to the growing phobia of death and physical decline and its links with the market, stressing its ethical and environmental significance and calling for a greater sense of responsibility towards the fundamental cultural issues. The resulting argument, deriving from my own personal involvement in the social and working context, will attempt to explain modern behaviour with ancient categories, through the language of the myths and symbols that unconsciously influence our language and our understanding. The evocative power of narrative can communicate a sense of the relativity of the real and suggest various things that could be changed. By *feeling* complexity, instead of just thinking about it, and by striving to go beyond specialization and automatism, to reach an intermediate space, an area of detachment from our own dominant attitudes, we can arrive at new possibilities.

'Necessary' repression

If the Greeks' rationality aimed at opening up a universe seen as a closed, delineated system, it still seemed to have an aesthetic basis (the Greek word *kosmos* meant 'ornament'). With the progressive replacement of nature by the inner human world, the presuppositions that made science possible were realized. The reification of nature, which today has led to our disregarding its rights and its beauty, has nevertheless produced, for the first time in the history of humankind, a kind of knowledge capable of formulating universal predicates. As Karl Popper,[1] and, in the medical field, Michel Foucault,[2] have shown, in contrast to ancient rationality, science develops in open systems and makes no claim today to reveal the secrets of existence, in the form of static 'truths'. It is sufficient to study a specific aspect of it, and to reveal particular 'secrets' in the form of mathematical predicates that are measurable and reproducible, and therefore 'universal'. This recognition of its intrinsic limitedness is a condition of the falsifiability of all scientific knowledge. Humility with regard to knowledge, however, is characteristic only of genuine scientists, such as Albert Einstein. Technology is different; it seems to have adopted the aspirations of ancient rationality in a concretistic manner, assuming titanic, neo-Promethean characteristics, in its alliance with economic and financial power. Medical technology, being truly able to prolong life, embodies a sense of power which is no longer merely practical but also metaphysical. In the face of the prospect of death and its complexity, the technological doctor embodies an immense power, that of exorcizing its terror and postponing its imminence. Consequently technology is burdened with a salvific projection which exposes human beings to the risk of a new inflation. A new, totalizing and individualizing view of the universe is subtly emerging, unconsciously realized in the present, instantaneous time of every technological operation and expressed by its capacity to modify existence, thus 'saving' life.

As described by the philosopher Jean-Luc Nancy,[3] in his reflections on the heart transplant that he underwent after severe heart failure, in the book *L'Intrus* ('The Intruder'), constantly postponing things to a non-time and a non-place puts the patient in the condition of spending a long time in a liminal zone of ambivalence between life and death, which, while revealing the indissoluble link between them, proves unacceptable and measureless to the human consciousness. Modern medicine risks condemning patients to a condition of being extraneous to themselves, because it makes them dependent on the constant intervention of *techne*. This dependence derives from the obligation to take medicines or from the indispensable use of biomedical devices, such as the modified or transplanted organ, a life-assisting machine device, or other interventions by healthcare technology. This produces a relative alienation of the ego, but also an ontological predominance of technical power over the patient: my ego is no longer under my control; it can no longer dispense with a will extraneous to it, which conditions its existence. The continual postponement of death underlines its imminence in an unnatural way and makes *repression* functionally useful. Avoiding a direct confrontation with the thought of death becomes necessary if one is to bear its unnatural burden on the consciousness. This, however, is not always possible, for example in people waiting for a heart transplant or in those who have an implantable cardioverter-defibrillator (ICD), two conditions where the incidence of depression, often with panic attacks, becomes particularly high. The reason is, in the former case, the fear of dying before a donor is found, and in the latter, the presence of an active 'intruder', the ICD, which emits a terrifying discharge in a completely unexpected and unpredictable manner; because it can recognize a threatening arrhythmia, its sudden electric shock literally saves your life. However, when this occurs quite frequently, as in the case of an arrhythmic storm, many patients are terrified.

Ironically, the metaphysical projection on to *techne* is destined to be eclipsed, both within the scientific paradigm itself and in the patient's psyche, at the moment of death, when everyone is finally obliged to accept its reality, which sometimes comes as a relief.

A new awareness on the part of operators, in the real world of medicine – not only in laboratories, lecture halls and narrow intellectual circles – can bring about change. The doctor can make the difference, by getting involved. The question is, how can we promote this awareness? It is not only patients who need to make the effort of *being* in the irrational dimension of existence, taking the time to listen to their own innermost feelings, with their subtle signals, their real or imagined symptoms, their unexpected dreams or diagnostic surprises, their prognostic doubts or existential problems, the tension of waiting or the disappointments, the hopes that unite or the sense of the inevitability of the end, and so on. If at certain moments we stop looking only at the great autonomous external reality of technological developments, we, both doctor and patient, can come into contact with ourselves. This sincere confrontation with existence on the part of many people transcends individuals, linking them together in a network of common humanity woven from the thin individuative[4] threads of everyone. This network makes a crucial contribution to the forces that extend history to include unheard and unspoken voices *across* time, developing a sense of a non-linear or meta-historical community of destiny. As a result of this ethical involvement, and the effort to be aware of their own complex inner and outer dimensions, both doctors and patients, while not denying the reality of evil and its inevitability, will not remain indifferent.[5]

Jung, interviewed in the late 1950s on the BBC programme *Face to Face*, stressed the psychic importance of death – the great existential weight that its inevitability implies at every moment.[6] The old psychoanalyst, his bright, youthful eyes shining throughout the interview, argued forcefully that we should always look forward, that we should *be* in life even when we are old; that we should avoid looking back, lest we risk, being turned to stone, like Lot in the Bible story. This effort is like a secular religiosity, which we can put into practice by resolving to be observant and attentive in our experience of *processes*. The aim of Part II of this book is to suggest that the reader should approach the experience of illness and its treatment in the same spirit.

In the face of the metaphysical unknown and the pragmatic doubt imposed by technology by the postponement of death, the doctor who accepts the fact of not knowing, and who chooses to engage his own subjective existence by listening, brings a sense of shared destiny and acceptance of chance to his solidarity with the patient. Openness to symbolic, intersubjective dialogue with patients and relatives, authentic listening, engagement in the intensity of particular moments, and attentive observation of processes, can help them to represent the prospect of death not as an end, but as a transition.[7]

The neurosis of life

The founding myth of medicine, its essential metaphor, is life. The contemporary concept of medicine, however, risks interpreting its mandate one-sidedly. This one-sidedness becomes evident, for example, in therapeutic persistence with the elderly, denial of their independence and reluctance to accept their death even when they have clearly reached the end. Experiences of profound denial of this kind are not uncommon, with difficulty in coming to terms with loss.[8] What is constantly denied through the various instances that are unconsciously projected is the psychic experience of death. This can even lead to the demonization and medicalization of suicide: there is a literal interpretation of the doctor's task as an agent of life, especially in the restricted meaning of organic life. The doctor is seen by one part of the public as the enactor and agent of a higher Apollonian and technological principle, capable of 'surgically' removing every symptom and illness and restoring patients, at any price, to their socially functional role, the *status quo ante*. Life, which in a wider sense includes death in every respect and is continually renewed by it, is interpreted in a narrow, dogmatic sense, driving the doctor's mandate to one-sidedness. It is important to understand how the obscurantist projections on to the doctor arise and stimulate each other. The doctor's attitude reinforces that of the patient and vice versa; this creates a vicious circle, reinforced by the external context of society and the family, and so it is possible to act on these conditionings only through an approach centred on the relationship.

James Hillman writes in *Suicide and the Soul*:

> *Organic death has absolute power over life when death has not been allowed in life's midst.* When we refuse the experience of death, we also refuse the essential question of life and leave life unaccomplished. Then

organic death prevents our facing the ultimate questions and cuts off our chance for redemption.[9]

One of the consequences is that at the moment of death in hospitals, acute patients often remain alone, their presence manifested only by the sounds of the machines to which they are connected until their last breath. Family members are deliberately kept away, temporarily protected from closeness to the dying person, and then confronted with the terror of loss when the naked vision of the corpse laid out in the pale attitude of death is restored to them. It is difficult, in the face of the anticipation of this terror, even to imagine an alternative to hospital treatment. It is becoming increasingly rare for patients to be given the choice of dying at home, without exposing themselves to strong resistance from their relatives, and sometimes even to a reduction in nursing care, for reasons of an economic or normative nature. Clinical care at home would require in such cases the implementation of special programmes and a varying degree of complexity. The statistics indicate that most deaths still occur in hospitals or nursing homes (though there is a gradual overall increase in hospice services to the elderly in the home setting).[10] Sometimes the ambulance services bring to hospitals the dead bodies of people of a very advanced age who have died at home to escape the total denial of relatives utterly incapable of accepting the impossibility of a life-saving operation or the irreversibility of the event, when the time for resuscitative manoeuvres is long past. In my experience, in cases which, by contrast, are recognized in time as particularly serious it has been possible to prepare the family for the possibility of giving the terminal patient a 'good death', and later keeping them company with renewed involvement, devotion and respect, even in the casualty ward of the hospital. But it is complicated, and very rare – though it reflects the wishes of many people, at least in Milan – to allow the family to take the dying person home. Sometimes the doctors and family members persuade the patient, often without meeting any resistance, to accept the risk of one final heroic endeavour, and they prefer to hope in a final apotropaic surgical gesture, which exorcizes death even for a short time, rather than accepting not only their loved one, but themselves and their own existential anguish.

The defensive reaction of the relatives, especially in cases of psychiatric illness, is well represented by Macbeth's request when confronted by the madness of Lady Macbeth. She is tormented by terrible visions of her guilt, which is irremediable because it is real. He asks the doctor if he cannot 'with some sweet oblivious antidote / cleanse the stuff'd bosom of that perilous stuff / which weighs upon the heart', as if he thought there might be a purely physical remedy and the burden of introspection could be avoided. When the doctor replies that it is precisely in that place, the heart, that the patient must 'minister to himself', he is met with denial and a paranoid reaction.[11]

Malcolm's approach to the suffering of the loyal MacDuff, when the latter receives the news that his wife and children have been slaughtered by Macbeth, is completely different. Even though this is a death by murder, not by disease, his words are extremely apposite to our case: 'give sorrow words. The grief that does not speak / Whispers the o'er fraught heart, and bids it break.'[12]

Today the illusion of the indefinite prolonging of organic life has created automatic expectations of a cure. The very limits of life have become ill defined. The boundary between life and death has become blurred, uncertain, pushed back beyond the death of the individual, for example by organ transplants. This leads to fantasies of life's infinite extendibility through such things as 'therapeutic' cloning, which concretizes the unconscious, atavistic longing for immortality.

What could be done, as an alternative, is to set up hospital units responsible for providing care at the homes of terminally ill elderly patients suffering from cancer or other diseases, should they decide, in agreement with their family, to forgo hospital treatment and return home. If this were possible, it would help to reduce the cost of providing care for people who occupy hospital beds for weeks, often in solitude; and at the same time it would offer a possibility of dignifying the relationship with death, by (re-)accepting the dying person – their body – as a reality and a presence, when the contingent conditions make it possible.

Repression of death and systemic waste: a 'cultural' cause of superfluity?

When we are struck by the certainty of illness, it is natural to flee from anything that points to the imminence of death: anything that brings it closer is ignored or repressed, because it is too greatly feared. But hidden within the tension of this defence may be the creative potential of the experience the psyche has of itself as the end draws near. This is probably even more the case in the present day: death has become the great repressed subject of our times, as has been mentioned above and extensively discussed by many authors.

Much of the administrative functioning of hospitals revolves around the interaction of this fundamental taboo of our age with the huge turnover of our profit-based society. The literal and one-sided interpretation of medicine's mandate, life, has been greatly stimulated by pseudo-ethical artifices and political masks, which are in fact complicit in the general frenzy of profiteering and try to create in the health sector yet another exploitable area of induced suffering and superfluous needs. The superabundance of investigations and operations in the last few decades has often been used more for calming the anxieties and fears of many patients than for real therapeutic purposes, but has continued to generate profit, at the expense of the welfare state and future generations. This incongruity is perceived particularly in the case of the elderly and the increasingly frequent chronically ill, with the spread of depression and psychosomatic illness.

The Slow Medicine movement has been conducting a campaign whose motto is 'Doing more does not mean doing better'; its exponents have succeeded in highlighting some highly important thematic areas, from the care of the elderly to palliative and end-of-life remedies, from health in reproduction and childhood to prevention and the promotion of healing, from the appropriateness of therapy to good communicative practice in the therapeutic relationship, from overmedicalization to conflict of interest and corruption, and finally to the need for a systemic vision in treatment. I came across the movement recently, and the reader is referred to their Italian (but multilingual) website www.slowmedicine.it for discussions of these subjects; it includes a considerable amount of audiovisual material by professionals from various backgrounds interested in raising public awareness of these issues.

The historian Eric Hobsbawm has described the interaction between culture and the globalized market in the following terms:

> From the point of view of the market, the only interesting culture is the product or service that makes money. But let us not be anachronistic. In the cultural fields the contemporary concept of 'the market' – an undiscriminating, globalising search for maximum profit – is quite novel [. . .] What is more, the concept of a single universal rate of profit to which all enterprise must conform is a recent product of the globalized free market, as is the concept that the sole alternative to going out of business is unlimited growth.[13]

To a certain extent this concept can be extended to include the absence of self-limitation in healthcare as well. The prevalence of the paradigms of individual interest, productivity and efficiency in the health sector has generated, with the corporatization of hospitals, a consumerist mentality in the medical sphere, based on the commercial exploitation of the repression of death. The denial and repression of the reality of illness and death, the absence of rites of passage and of a collective imagination of the end of life are, at least in part, the origin of the massive demand for healthcare. The counterpart is a return of the repressed in the form of a neurosis about good health and a massive medicalization of society, quantifiable in terms of the number of services provided, and stimulated by the colossal private profits of the multinationals, which gain from public healthcare (pharmaceutical companies, firms that produce biomedical technologies, medical equipment, services, etc.). The paradoxical effect is that the logic of efficiency and targets finds itself contributing indirectly to an enormous 'systemic healthcare wastage', masked by supposed objectivity and technicism.[14]

Lastly, there is another consequence of the spread of 'functionalism' in the age of technology: the defensiveness of medicine. In the context of the increasing hypertrophy of rules and regulations and the weakening of the family, which is unwilling or unable to look after the sick person, doctors 'arm' themselves with numerous precautions, with a further excess of services. A population with an increasingly high average age will continue to demand passively from health authorities an immediate response to their high expectations of treatment and will not easily accept that the doctor might disappoint them.

There is therefore a link between a demand for healthcare driven beyond all reasonable bounds (well beyond the 'needs' whose inviolability has been at the heart of many political programmes), and the mechanisms of capitalist accumulation. This problem, which goes beyond the question of the appropriateness of the treatments, is connected with the creation of a large and constantly growing population of patients with multiple chronic conditions, comprising the 'survivors' of acute conditions, the heirs of death postponed thanks to the extreme therapeutic efficacy of empirical medicine in the acute context. These patients are heavily dependent on hospital care for their continued survival. Facing up to this problem involves the need to create the necessary space and to accept within the administrative paradigm cultural and psychological factors, which administrators too perhaps begin to become aware of when they are faced with the problem of handling those suffering from serious chronic conditions and the problem of the end of life.[15]

The mythology of everyday life

In this chapter we will examine some 'myths' of our age and the denied opposite that they can represent in the medical field, conditioning both the 'health operative' and the public comprising patients and their relatives – that is, in practice (sooner or later) the whole of society. As with every unconscious one-sided decision, there is a conversion into the opposite, as a return of the repressed. The term *enantiodromia*, originally from Heraclitus (it is derived from *enantios*, 'opposite', and *dromos*, 'running'), means literally 'a running counter to', and was adopted by Jung; this phenomenon 'practically always occurs when an extreme, one-sided tendency dominates conscious life; in time an equally powerful counterposition is built up, which first inhibits the conscious performance and subsequently breaks through the conscious control.'[16]

To this Jung adds an observation which indicates the route to a solution:

The only person who escapes the grim law of enantiodromia is the man who knows how to separate himself from the unconscious, not repressing it – for then it simply attacks him from the rear – but *by putting it clearly before him as that which he is not.*[17]

The constant denial of physical decline and therefore, in the final instance, of death generates an immense market of aesthetic surgery operations, cosmetic products, tattoos, body-building, health-consciousness, hygiene concerns and superfluous medicines. The medicalization of psychic suffering – a drug for every ailment, however minor – combines with the standardization of the relationship with the corporeal, thanks in part to representations by the media, advertising and fashion. If the denial of death is not directly 'enacted' on a person's objectualized body, it is in any case filtered through the collective imagination's fixation with advertising, which invades the subjective sphere through the mass media.

As has already been mentioned, a metaphysics of science and a heroism of technological human beings become a formidable tool at the service of a grandiosity of action, which must – always, and whatever the situation – defeat or eliminate the illness. Medicine's mandate, life, becomes one-sided, and the denial of the inner evil (sickness and demonized death) may be transformed into a gigantism of the human being. In the same way the expectations of a cure – or of 'being put back into working order' – on the part of patients (who in return agree to be treated as objects) become virtually absolute. This leads to a vicious circle of legislative hypertrophy, a cause of a further excess of treatments, hospitalizations, operations and so on.

The bulimia of the health market is sustained by 'new' myths, which can all be traced back to the denial of limits (and hence, in the final instance, of death), which have caused a progressive medicalization of society.

In the first place, there is the *obsession with looking young at all costs*, and therefore the *denial of old age.* This leads to numerous activities designed to prove the contrary. For example, the excesses of plastic surgery: external beauty as a surrogate for eternal youth – not as an innate internal image: an old person's wrinkles tell the story of that person's life, yet the canon of television beauty is a mirror distorted by the fear of physical deterioration. The values of old age – experience, wisdom, knowledge of the world, but also slowness, reflectiveness, the paradoxical availability of time, essentiality – are devalued, and old people themselves are at risk of interiorizing the youthful model of hyperactivity, to give themselves and others the impression that they are still young. The wrinkles erased from the face, the stretched skin, swollen lips and stereotyped nose of some caricatural faces try to concretize in the form sculpted by the surgeon the projective image of TV programmes and advertisements, but contain the tragic nemesis of the events that have informed their creation.

Another 'myth', which manifests itself as 'implicit', a pervasive and contagious manner capable of conditioning behaviour, consists of the urgency of a rapid satisfaction of needs. The *inability to postpone needs* determines an extreme facility in the medicalization of the symptom; for example, the indiscriminate use of painkillers, antibiotics and anxiolytics, and homoeopathic remedies (for even homoeopathic medicine is not immune to this concept), especially in the treatment of children, with a consequent medicalization of society, systemic waste and difficulty in disposing of huge amounts of medicinal refuse. Every ailment, however minor, requires an immediate remedy. The commercial exploitation of this urgency leads to the carrying out of diagnostic tests and surgical operations even when they are not strictly necessary, in order to banish an irrational anxiety about waiting, which is seen as something unbearable.

An important element in determining the mechanism of treatment is a *mythology of 'doing'* – that is, doing more and more – whereby the doctor becomes a human prosthesis of the interests of *techne*, incapable of imagining his own or the patient's freedom. Allied to this is a relative invisibility of the fruits of reflective observation, of time spent waiting – in contrast to what used to happen in the *temenos* – but also a loss of the long-term view which has an effect on cultural and behavioural conditionings which cause illness: for example, a therapeutic or surgical medicine in contrast to a cognitive or preventive one. Often the surgical short-cut is preferred to medical alternatives, for example in the failure to face up to the socio-cultural problem of infantile obesity – whose origins can be traced back to the preschool, and even the pre-natal period[18] – and the bulimia which underlies it, and the consequent use of bariatric surgery even on young patients.

The grandiosity and 'unpostponability' of action underlines the problem of the appropriateness of treatment and too easily removes not only the question of sustainability but also that of the health consequences of rampant consumerism, and particularly of widespread overeating. The antithesis of sobriety – food addiction, or obesity – may be grouped with other addictions (smoking, alcohol, medicine, sex and drugs). Counterposed to them, at the other end of the spectrum, is the utopia of absolute prevention, an exclusive belief in the values of Hygieia.

At a level more specifically linked to the psychological attitude of doctors, and so strong as sometimes to risk conditioning their moral integrity, is the *myth of work as the hypostasis of 'success'*. This manifests itself in the prioritizing of work over life and consequently in the loss of the human dimension of work and a further dehumanization and de-individuation of the individual. The quest for subjectivity and for a realization of the 'fundamentally human' seem not to find any place or to withdraw increasingly from working hours and the workplace, impoverishing the latter by depriving it of its greatest resource – individual creativity. Aristotle's *praxis* works as an end in itself; action with a view to *philia* – relationship or proximity – and education, is inevitably replaced by result-oriented *poiesis* ('making'), the daughter of *techne* and objectifying reason; it pursues self-perfection as its sole aim, with a view to production, irrespective of the patient. It is indicative that today the noun 'practice', in the sense of being practical, appears to have inverted its etymological meaning. Nevertheless, the tension between the two phases forms a constituent, structural and in this sense necessary feature of the complexity of contemporary medical work – which is such that one cannot entirely opt for it either by the logic of the stick and carrot or by that of the inner motivators alone. Moreover, families are weakened too, for when creativity finds no outlet in work, the search for Eros will take other paths, characterized by instability of feeling, paths which cannot replace work as an environment of self-fulfilment. The statistics for separation and divorce show that they are particularly frequent in the medical profession.

The central myth is that of *power*, because of what I have called the 'Asclepius complex', which manifests itself as *omnipotence in the face of death* – omnipotence concealed in altruism, sometimes unconsciously enacted, but sometimes conscious: doctors, embodying the power of science and technology, feed on it and contribute to the progressive medicalization of society. Doctors who pretend that they know more than they really do, that they alone have the right remedy for every condition and for the largest number of patients. Doctors who set out to identify with patients' projections but who never reveal to them the emotional origin of their ailments, and do not even touch on the tragic reality of the social and human context that every life expresses in its recourse to help. Professionals who do not exercise their cognitive interest in the environmental complexity, of which they could become valuable critics and observers, thanks to the window that society offers them. Doctors who are motivated by an aggressive or indifferent unconscious dimension, which reveals that the patient's destiny is of little interest to them. Lastly, cynics, who do their work with detachment, and paradoxically prove less harmful than some doctors who feel a need for confirmation or identify with the ultimate aims of science. People who, under the pretext of pressure of time, act out their own shadow, perhaps behind a smug smile, and keep their involvement to the minimum. Or they exploit a trusting or submissive attitude in some patients, to give free rein to their inclinations, prescribing or carrying out invasive manoeuvres. People who listen only superficially, faced with a large number of patients complaining of vague symptoms, and who only apply criteria of epidemiological probability. The patients will be examined from head to foot and subjected to numerous diagnostic tests and operations whose usefulness is doubtful to say the least, giving full consent to their medicalization and pathologicization. The patients will obtain, through the direct modification of their body – the so-called 'organic substratum' – an illness that they did not have before (the after-effects of an operation). The demand for resolutive, relief-bringing aid constitutes a strong and constant stimulus to Asclepius's constellation of the shadow. The role of the charlatan is sometimes consciously adopted for money-making purposes, and in this case the doctors practise their profession in total identification with their shadow, more for their own advantage than with a real intention of providing assistance and a cure.

The foundation of a balance that can avoid constellating the brutality of power on the part of the doctor is precisely the uncertainty of the result and a certain neutrality which admits shadows, a fundamental honesty with oneself and willingness to acknowledge one's own mistakes. When the diagnosis becomes a death sentence and any therapy an atonement, any possibility of Eros comes to be circumscribed within the power complex, which is its exact opposite. As Jung stated:

> Logically the opposite of love is hate, and of Eros, Phobos (fear); but psychologically it is the will to power. Where love rules, there is no will to power, and where power predominates, love is lacking. The one is the shadow of the other.[19]

The market, and money, deserve separate consideration. The market as financial power not subjected to controls by powers external to it, the capitalism of profit and unlimited growth, will account for millions of superfluous operations in hospitals every year. The shadow of Hermes, the spirit of commerce, a mischievous, wily thief, beloved of Zeus, still winks at us from the bank vaults, from the microchips of the stock-market flows, from behind the movements of oil, gas, arms and drugs and their lowest common denominator, money-laundering, as well as the channels of tax avoidance. Where money stops, we can rediscover value. Probably the places where it is most concentrated could supply the founding metaphor of modern 'sanctity' and unlimited desire.

The market, and money, cannot be judged by the same criteria as the previous categories. They are structural factors, whose symbolic function depends on the complex web of signifiers embedded in the power relations of society as a whole. So it is worth dwelling on this point a little longer, though the subject is a vast one.

In a world infinitely rich in projections manipulated by the media, where the projective channels and their dynamisms represent the 'highways' of libidinal desires, countless networks of compulsive ties are created, based on the expectations projected on to objects. They are the unlived lives, the other great consequence of repressed death. In this context, the libidinal investment moves progressively from concrete objects to the money that can acquire everything. Money becomes the simulacrum of a universal and final receptacle of a libidinal energy that has become impersonal. By virtue of the importance that is attached to it, as a guarantor of all the chains of compulsive relationships, it becomes the very place of life and action. Vast energies move along the axes of the desiring projections banished to a fetishist and literalist imagination. The vital energy is all the more linked to money, the less the individual is capable of developing an inner dimension, rich in autonomous vital images. The individual will have difficulty in achieving independence from the absolute importance attributed to the external object. Sex and money go together because they function as a surrogate for the lack of Eros in life. The central value of the immediate satisfaction of (repressed) desire/(induced) need is associated with the *myth of eternal youth* and the *mythicizing of the body*.

This is sometimes accompanied by a utopia of the beauty and speed of the technological object. This is revealed partly in the passion many doctors have for electronic products, the desire for which fills our psyche and creates a kind of buffer space, an in-between area, a perimetral 'no-fly zone', around which is constructed the ideal of the robotized apartment (home automation) and of the garage with an electric shutter, all combined with the aerodynamic elegance of the sports car or the more compact style of the off-roader. But both ironically find their mechanical nemesis in the great metropolitan road congestion: drivers find themselves alone in their cars, distracted by the company of a radio, separated in space, and yet united via the ether by the accelerating patter of TV news broadcasts and adverts.

The current model of growth could destroy the earth in a short time if it were applied to the whole of living humanity in constant demographic increase. An obvious example is the economic expansion of the BRICS (Brazil, Russia, India, China and South Africa). Even more significant is the urbanization and current capitalist development of China.

All over the globe, the model seems to be the same, the universal goal or 'common home' of the bourgeois ideal, cutting across every creed and ethnic origin, whose supremacy is mediated today especially by the image and comfort, not by conceptual content, and whose authoritativeness is based on its never-ending and unstoppable reproduction and diffusion. This model exerts a constant pressure, asserted through the laws of the market, with the increasingly competitive prices of industrial production. In this way it removes every new obstacle to the diffusion of technological functionalism and facilitates the penetration of its consumerist, utilitarian social equivalent. The great mass of the *Lumpenproletariat*, of those excluded from the Internet economy, remains available for work. Today this great human reservoir represents the real fuel and at the same time the weak link in the economic hyperbole, as well as an immense market for medicine: participating in global competitiveness because it has no choice but to supply its labour at a low cost, it promotes the growth of the bourgeoisie on a global scale, both inside its own country and outside it, through the great ongoing migrations or the widespread dispersal of the places of production of the various industries. This phenomenon is linked to a process of growing difference in wealth on a planetary scale which is causing a downgrading of the social pact and welfare in the West.

One only has to think of the vast number of home helps and carers in the world of paramedical assistance. Or of the competitive prices for services whose added value is marked down, without there being any substantial loss in the quality of the product or the service provided (for example, medical, dental or beauty treatment, provided by immigrant staff or located on the margins of developed areas). Or – and this is particularly important – of the potential for sales of know-how, services and medical technologies in the process of medicalization of entire societies in the developing and less consumerized countries. What are the implications in terms of social cost and pollution (medical X-rays are an important source of radioactive waste), and how will the relationship with nature and death change in these populations?

Is it possible that the appetite of the masses included in the historical process through industrial production and consumption will one day reach the limit of sustainability – that nausea and fear will become global? No one can say for sure. Perhaps the scenario will change, and, by doing so, transform the language and concept of well-being, but these questions are still open. All this is the effect of a great transition, an epochal transformative tension, whose extremes appear to us dichotomously because of the enormity of the conflict that is in progress, but they are also beyond our capacity for comprehension, because we are part of them and we are experiencing day by day their possibilities and effects.

Inflation in the age of technology is not of human beings; it seems to be of objects, or rather of human beings made inseparable from their technological extensions, to which they run the risk of selling their souls, but which they can't do without; they project their soul and genius on to them, and invest their vital energy in them, but in their presence they run the risk of becoming dehumanized or being reduced to the passiveness of 'disposability'.

The fulcrum of this subject revolves around the market as the last residual domain of the transpersonal, so volatile as almost entirely to elude the examination of criticism and dialectic, but capable by contrast of commodifying thought. The globalized world seems to revolve around an area of the psyche which combines the tenacity and adaptability of the historic heritage of centuries of mercantilism (and thriving of the bourgeoisie) with the originally puritan concept of the irrational: the mad, unchangeable and admirable intransigence of egoic determination ('admirable' because of the selective advantage it offers in the fight for survival). The assumption of many supporters of concretism is fundamentally optimistic and anti-psychological. One must maintain a positive conception of one's identity *come what may*, even without a reflective process renewing it and being able to integrate its dark sides. It seems that thought pays the price of an ancient conditioning, that of the immensity of the energy and sacrifice expended by human beings down the centuries in order to survive; the memory of that effort, made superfluous by technological comfort, can generate a significant 'libidinal surplus' and be reinvested in an indefinite expansion of power, turning into mania. The *folle volo* ('mad flight') is no longer that of Ulysses,[20] but that of Captain Ahab; his is the metaphor of great love for the 'wilderness', which provides an explanation for the violence of history and lays the foundation for the commodification of the world, making deterministic the acceptance of its price at a human and natural level, as if it were the least of evils. Ahab is fulfilled, whatever the cost – even the final self-sacrifice for the sake of capturing and killing Moby Dick. He will die seemingly happy, gripping the harpoon rammed into the back of the whale, which drags him, his body maimed, down towards death, towards the nothingness of the sea and its depths.

However, the commodification of the world has today become a reality. Moreover, the exact sciences have reached such a degree of complexity as to be sometimes incomprehensible, often remote and inaccessible. So on this basis one could delineate, in place of the market and money and in contraposition to the ideological tensions described above, some *positive 'myths' of globalization*, of sociological derivation, which are, unlike those mentioned earlier, intrinsic to science itself and its realizations, and as such endowed with a great power of self-transformation in reality. A systematic discussion of this subject would go beyond the scope of this text; so I will simply refer the reader for further details to the relevant sociological literature, especially Manuel Castells's *The Rise of the Network Society*.[21]

Let us consider some of these new 'myths'. In the first place there is the 'hypertext' created by the net – the World-Wide Web – linking every possible narrative, past, present and future, in a single neutral time, which is beyond all possibility of comprehension, constantly shifting its frame of reference. Its negative aspect is the elimination of the past, and therefore of history as memory: the way it impedes the painstaking creation of a collective narrative, as if life could be conceived only abstractly, by continual pursuit of an artificial but alien future. It is important to note that, as has already been mentioned, the hypertext entails a cognitive standardization arising from the medium itself, and that the net society is characterized by a pervasive dynamic expansion which gradually absorbs and suppresses all pre-existent social forms. This can expand into a protean movement of capital to commodify and/or destroy all forms of life for the sake of profit. A further corollary, in the neo-liberalist sense, is the *self-regulation of free systems*, culminating in the denial of the nation state (a silent form of global re-territorialization), whose functions are ultimately transferred to a global economic oligarchy; the local hyper-nationalisms and populisms of the present day are an alienated reaction to this which attempt to recreate invented identities, often of a neo-pagan nature. The foundational characteristics of the myth are *individuality*, as opposed to dynamic relation, and *interactivity* mediated exclusively by the 'web'.[22] Its economic correlates are *competitivity* and *productivity*, in the context of a global interdependence realized through the universality of debt and the consequent imperative of connectivity, infrastructural development and growth. The individual is capitalized as a body deprived of its multi-organ complexity which is deemed to be solely responsible for the functioning of the system and is therefore subject to economic sanctions and deterrence. The circulation of capital is global, but the circulation of work is not; the spread of organized crime is global, but that of governance is not. *The relationship between debt and desire has become structural*, thus shaping and delimiting subjectivities, depriving the imaginal of potentiality and defining the 'real'.

There is also a technological widening of the biological field, which is increasingly conceived of in a cognitive way: the biogenetic revolution and the biotechnologies have 'truly' given science the power of ontologically changing reality; would Nietzsche ever have imagined that the original aspiration of science – that of reaching the heart of being and even changing it – would, in a sense, become reality in this field? Then there is the infinite *calculatio* associated with an almost unlimited, and profoundly anti-Platonic, expansion of memory, with the use of megadata, the idea of security based on the storing of intercepted data on a global scale (the NSA, or National Security Agency), the constantly changing calculations on which the great gambling den of finance is based, with its concentric levels of probability calculation with a view to maximizing profits, something possible on this scale only in the financial sphere. Austerity policies are based on highly complex models of real-time debt calculations which are never called into question and tend to escape scrutiny in the public domain.

Thus – to come to the possible symbolic meaning of the elements discussed above – according to the narrative set out in Part I, humankind has finally acquired the divine attributes of *omnipotence* (unlimited energy, nuclear power, technology), *omnipresence* (the ubiquity and 'portableness' of the web) *omniscience* (the hypertext) and *ability to create* (genetic engineering).

Notes

1 Popper 1934–1959.
2 Foucault 1963.
3 Nancy 2000.
4 As opposed to being deterministically individualized – a term used by Michel Foucault – through external systemic factors.
5 Cf. Neumann 1948 and Levi 1947. In the first text, written in 1943, the author shows how an authentic ethical position is possible at an individual level if one makes a constant effort to differentiate one's own consciousness from the regressive influence of the group. The tendency of the old ethics, derived from the traditional monotheisms is that of judging the evil and eliminating it without any mediation, condemning it with an unreflecting action that admits of no doubts. This will lead to the identification and 'expulsion' of a culprit according to the logic of the scapegoat, to redeem the group and restore it to a state of original purity. Traditional dogmatic ethics denies the existence of evil and conceives of it as an absence of the good (*privatio boni*). Furthermore, Levi (p. 9):

> Many, both individuals and peoples, may come to believe, more or less consciously, that 'every foreigner is an enemy'. For the most part this conviction lies in the depths of minds like a latent infection; it manifests itself only in periodic, uncoordinated acts, and is not the origin of a system of thought. But when this happens, when the unexpressed dogma becomes the major premise of a syllogism, then the concentration camp is at the end of the chain.

6 Jung 1959, interview.
7 Renz 2012.
8 Kübler Ross 1969.
9 Hillman 1965, p. 62.
10 Cf. websites: Teno 2013 and see also Dudgeon 1995.
11 Shakespeare, *Macbeth*, Act V, Scene III, lines 39–48: '*Macbeth*. Cure of that. / Canst thou not minister to a mind diseas'd, / Pluck from the memory a rooted sorrow, / Raze out the written troubles of the brain, / And with some sweet oblivious antidote / Cleanse the stuff'd bosom of that perilous stuff / Which weighs upon the heart? / *Doctor*. Therein the patient / Must minister to himself. / *Macbeth*. Throw physics to the dogs. I'll none of it. / Come, put mine armour on; give me my staff.'
12 Ibidem, Act IV, Scene III, lines 209–210.
13 Hobsbawm 2013, p. 48.
14 I give the data of the Institute of Medicine of Washington D.C. on the situation of federal American healthcare: in an article titled *The Health Care Imperative: Lowering Costs and Improving Outcomes* the amount of annual systemic wastage is estimated at about $765 billion, a sum equivalent to about 30% of the entire federal healthcare expenditure, about half of which is linked to superfluous

or inefficient treatment (see Institute of Medicine 2010). It has been estimated that problems like poor treatment quality, excess of therapy and administrative waste account for $1 trillion per year in costs that do not contribute to any improvement in the health of the population (see Berwick 2011). With this kind of sums it would be theoretically possible to solve some fundamental problems of the human race as a whole. If current laws and practices continue, health expenditures in the United States by the year 2030, as America's baby boomers enter their seventies and eighties, will top $16 trillion, or 32 per cent of GDP (see Burner 1992).

15 In 2001, 5 per cent of the beneficiaries of Medicare – the US health institution responsible for the care of elderly – received 43 per cent of the overall expenditure of the American health system, and 25 per cent of the patients accounted for 85 per cent of the total expenditure! (see Websites, Congressional Budget Office 2005). Three quarters of these patients have one or more chronic conditions; a key factor in the inefficiency is identified as the lack of co-ordinated treatments that could keep patients out of hospitals (see Fineberg 2012).

16 Jung 1921, p. 426.

17 Jung 1953, p. 73; the italics are in the original text.

18 Wojcicki 2010.

19 Jung 1953, p. 53.

20 Dante Alighieri, *Inferno*, XXVI, 125.

21 These recent 'myths' bring me to another point, that of 'branding' and the quest for an identity. Identity is related to culture, and culture is related to searching, and therefore implies that time is needed for reflection, a long time (which we do not usually grant ourselves). This is particularly so when we think of the contemporary perception that time is accelerating. I therefore have thought of developing in this book not a dichotomy, but rather a theoretical distinction between culture, understood as a process, a quest for identity, and civilization, in the sense of a technological, functional, acquired heritage. And this brings us to the crucial issue – the relationship between the local and the global dimensions. The quest for identity is related to the domain of individual existence, and is dissociated from what philosophers would call the domain of the exercise of power, which is global. Thus, the link between ordinary people and the political authorities, between the individual context and the collective one, needs deeper reflection, and the person who creates the sign, the simulacrum, the brand, must have a certain degree of awareness, for there are ethical aspects to the discussion. Starting from that point, we can go ahead and forge a discourse that distinguishes between the identity research process, linked to a particular place, and the hypertext, which belongs to the Internet. The *hypertext*, originally a sociological term coined by Manuel Castells in the previously mentioned book 'The rise of the network society' – that is, of the World Wide Web – blends all possible past, present and future narratives into an eternal present-day one. This creates a division, a dichotomy, where every imaginable tale has already been told and will be present for all eternity. This must be borne in mind, for it entails a cognitive systematic homologation taken from the medium itself: the medium is not neutral (Marshall McLuhan), and the network society is characterized by a dynamic and pervasive expansion, which gradually absorbs and subordinates all previous social forms. So narrative becomes something insubstantial; it cannot be extrapolated from the individual context. It is in an attempt to deal with this problem that Mark Zuckerberg has purchased a gigantic drone to carry the Internet to tribal populations in remote parts of the globe. Mega-data artificial intelligence technologies have been used to create simplified low-cost mobile phones that turn

spoken words into texts, so that populations with oral traditions and an ancient sense of identity will be connected to Facebook and the web. And this is just one example of what the above-mentioned divide might become. In this respect, there is some interesting evidence of the historical connection between branding and psychoanalysis. The counterculture of the 1960s came as a shock to the business corporations, which dissociated themselves from it. Later, however, they realized that they needed to assimilate the psychoanalytical concepts involved. This was precisely the time when some minor figures connected with Freud, such as Edward Bernays, contributed to the invention of advertising, public relations and marketing; it was the age of the birth of the simulacrum. Images rather than products, desire rather than need. In a society in which basic needs are satisfied, a psychic overflow arose, so business corporations sought to induce a dependence on the external object. Ernest Dichter, who came to be known as the Freud of Madison Avenue, talked of the therapeutic power of consumption. Products became psychological extensions of the consumer's identity; *the object's expressive power was actually extended to include loyalty to the commercial brand, and this was interpreted as loyalty to oneself*. This greatly increased the complexity of the search for identity in post-modern society. Branding began at a time when the first focus groups were being created, beginning with group therapy and psychoanalytical work. All this illustrates the risk, at both the technological and the political levels, of the 'outsourcing' of the soul to the concrete object of desire. Thus part of the psyche ends up conforming to the market in its search for identity. That is, the risk of developing a commodified false self, leading to short-lived and 'ready-made' identities, which would change continually and would therefore struggle to reach a deeper level of understanding. On the other hand, the web might also provide, especially for technologically and culturally qualified individuals, a widening horizon, that is, a widening of horizons from the local to the global that may open the way to unforeseeable and unknown development.

22 Before the era of information technology, Pier Paolo Pasolini, in declaring his love for tradition, for the past and for history, already placed himself on the side of the 'excluded', that is to say, of that *Lumpenproletariat* which has never entered the consumer society and is still not part of the present-day 'online' society. The world of economic exclusion sanctioned by proprietary right, the world of hunger and exclusion, numbers about 2 billion people today, including a large number of tribal populations in different continents and the great urban pockets of the metropolises of the whole globe. Their exclusion is an exclusion from attention, from memory and from history. Pasolini also spoke of 'a new prehistory, which is dawning for the bourgeois world, the world of technology, and the world of neo-capitalism' and nostalgia for the sacred and for ancient values, where a longing for the past is accepted as a conservative emotion (see Pasolini 1962).

Bibliography

Berwick, Donald M. (2011), *The Moral Test*: Speech at the Institute for Health Care Improvement National Forum, Orlando FL, 7/12/2011. www.ihi.org/resources/Pages/AudioandVideo/Don-Berwick-Forum-Keynotes.aspx Accessed 30th October 2017.

Burner, Sally T. et al. (1992), 'National Health Expenditures Projections through 2030', *Health Care Financing Review*, 14, Part 1 (1992), pp. 1–29.

Castells, Manuel (1996), *The Rise of the Network Society: The Information Age, Vol. 1: Economy, Society and Culture*, Oxford: Blackwell Publishers, 1996.

Congress of the United States, Congressional Budget Office, 'High-Cost Medicare Beneficiaries', A CBO Paper, May 2005. www.cbo.gov/sites/default/files/cbofiles/ftpdocs/63xx/doc6332/05-03-medispending.pdf Accessed 11th November 2017.

Dudgeon, Deborah et al. (1995), 'Home versus Hospital Death: Assessment of Preferences and Clinical Challenges', *Canadian Medical Association Journal*, 152.3 (1995), p. 337. www.cmaj.ca/content/152/3/337 Accessed 30th October 2017.

Fineberg, Harvey V. (2012), 'A Successful and Sustainable Health System: How to Get There from Here', *New England Journal of Medicine*, 366 (2012), pp. 1020–1027.

Foucault, Michel (1963), *Naissance de la Clinique. The Birth of the Clinic: An Archaeology of Medical Perception*, translated by Alan Mark Sheridan, London: Tavistock, 1976 [c. 1973].

Hillman, James (1965), *Suicide and the Soul*, Putnam, CT: Spring Publications, 1997.

Hobsbawm, Eric (2013), 'Politics and Culture in the New Century: Hesse Lecture at the Aldeburgh Festival' (2002), in *Fractured Times: Culture and Society in the Twentieth Century*, New York: The New Press, 2013.

Institute of Medicine (USA) (2010), 'The Healthcare Imperative: Lowering Costs and Improving Outcomes', Workshop Series Summary', in *Roundtable on Evidence-Based Medicine*, edited by P.L. Yong, R.S. Saunders, and L.A. Olsen, Washington, DC: National Academies Press, 2010. www.nap.edu/catalog/12750.html Accessed 30th October 2017.

Jung, Carl Gustav (1921), *Psychologische Typen, Psychological Types*, Bollingen Series XX, Vol. 9, Part I of the Collected Works of C.G. Jung, A revision by Richard Francis Carrington Hull of the translation by Helton Godwin Baynes, Princeton, NJ: Princeton University Press, 1971.

Jung, Carl Gustav (1953), *Zwei Schriften über Analytische Psychologie. Two Essays on Analytical Psychology*, Bollingen Series XX, Vol. 7 of the Collected Works of C.G. Jung, translated by Richard Francis Carrington Hull, London & New York: Routledge, 1990.

Jung, Carl Gustav (1959), Face to Face Interview [BBC – 1959]. www.youtube.com/watch?v=eTBs-2cloEI Accessed 30th October 2017.

Kübler Ross, Elisabeth (1969), *On Death and Dying: What the Dying Have to Teach Doctors, Nurses, Clergy and Their Own Families*, New York: Scribner, 2014.

Levi, Primo (1947), *Se Questo è un Uomo*, Turin: Einaudi, 2005.

Nancy, Jean-Luc (2000), *L'intrus*, Paris: Galilée, 2010; published in English as the last chapter of *Corpus*, translated by Richard A. Rand, New York: Fordham University Press, 2008, pp. 161–170.

Neumann, Erich (1948), *Tiefenspsychologie und Neue Ethic. Depth Psychology and a New Ethic*, translated by Eugene Rolfe, Boston & London: Shambala, 1990.

Pasolini, Pier Paolo (1962), 'Risposta a un Insoddisfatto', *Vie nuove*, 22 November, 1962.

Popper, Karl (1934–59), *Logik der Forschung* (1935). *The Logic of Scientific Discovery* (1959), London & New York: Routledge, 1992.

Renz, Monika et al. (2012), 'Dying Is a Transition', *American Journal of Hospice and Palliative Medicine*, 30.3 (July 12, 2012), pp. 283–290. https://doi.org/10.1177/1049909112451868 Accessed 30th October 2017.

Teno, Joan M. et al. (2013), 'Change in End-of-Life Care for Medicare Beneficiaries: Site of Death, Place of Care, and Health Care Transitions in 2000, 2005 and 2009', *Journal of the American Medical Association*, 309, part 5 (2013), pp. 470–477. www.ncbi.nlm.nih.gov/pmc/articles/PMC3674823/ Accessed 30th October 2017.

Wojcicki, Janet M. & Heyman, Melvin B. (2010), 'Let's Move: Childhood Obesity Prevention from Pregnancy and Infancy Onward', *New England Journal of Medicine*, 362, part 16 (April 22, 2010), pp. 1457–1459. www.nejm.org/doi/full/10.1056/NEJMp1001857 Accessed 30th October 2017.

Chapter 4

Narcissus's mirror

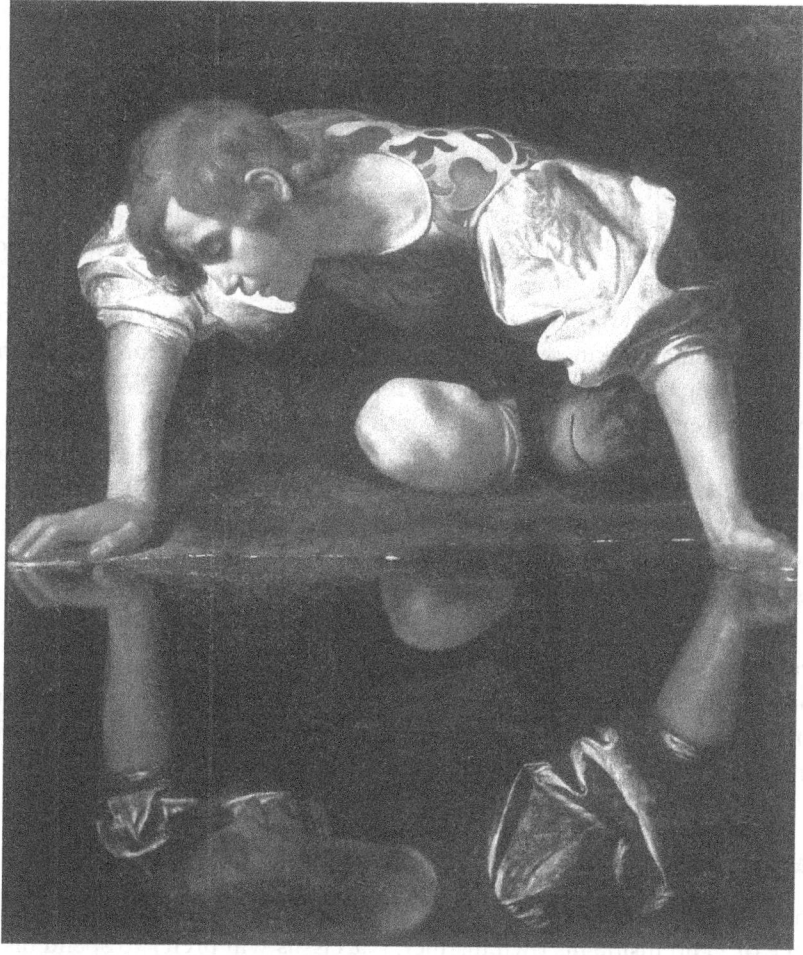

Figure 4.1 Caravaggio's *Narcissus* (1594–96). In the public domain, Galleria Nazionale d'Arte
Antica, Palazzo Barberini, Rome.

Scan – Wikimedia Commons.

The following observations on Narcissism are made with the aim of investigating the psychological motivations that favour the development of present-day consumeristic bulimia, both in medicine and in contemporary western society as a whole. A deeper knowledge of the widespread Narcissistic tendency in our society helps us understand the omnipotent inclination of the attitude of doctors and patients, with implications that are both ethical – affecting the ways in which medicine is practised – and quantitative – because of the risk of a hypermedicalization of society. The medicalizing factor depends on the distorted perception of the psychological function of medicine with respect to the symptom in the collective context. A medicine preoccupied with 'removing evil' becomes functional to the expectations of a society made up of relatively undifferentiated individuals, less able to accept difficulties extraneous to their Narcissistic self-referentialism. Illness often comes as a compensation for this one-sided attitude and appears unexpectedly, when Narcissus encounters his own image and in so doing perishes.

In Caravaggio's representation of Narcissus (see Figure 4.1), the reflected image is not identical to Narcissus's face in the daylight, especially in the colours, made darker and less distinct by the depth of the water. The face is bluish in the shadow; the expression too seems tinged with melancholy, the eyes drooping and tired, the face gaunt, lined with wrinkles, worn not by age but by suffering, or perhaps by illness. The painting suggests at first sight the intimate connection between this 'mirroring' and the snares inherent in relating to one's own 'shadow', reflected in the ego's mirror. Narcissus appears never to have noticed this dark nuance in the face with which he had 'fallen' in love until this precise moment. There seems to have been, as a condition of his falling in love, an omission, a subtle denial – preconscious, but still close to the field of intentionality – which alone makes passionate attraction possible, by remaining on the surface. The self-healing nature of this attraction is directed, however, not at the real object, but unconsciously towards that same dark, mysterious object, behind which the fragile, vulnerable personality of the narcissist lies hidden. Here the artist depicts the moment that precedes the discovery of the deception; in seeking physical contact with the reflection, Narcissus discovers that it was in fact a projection of himself.

Narcissus and the shadow

Whereas Pan, in the exuberance of his desire, accepts the reflection of the image of Echo inside his own instinct, Narcissus will prefer to spend his life at the mirror. He is not rooted in instinct; Echo is unequivocally rejected by him, just as his instinctual nature is repressed. He will refuse to set any limits to his own desire, which for this very reason will never be satisfied. The object, being an ideal object, will always be referred to the external mirror, where Narcissus ultimately will not be able to help unconsciously projecting himself. So narcissism is profoundly anti-tragic and linked to the shadow of our age.

'In these mists of time Narcissus still lives, wounded by a mirror, which was not water, but glass.' This short line of poetry, written by a young adult at the beginning of his analysis, seems to suggest a modern variant of the ancient myth. Narcissus never dies, because he never meets his image in the water, but in the fragile glass, which conceals no depth.

Narcissus, in Ovid's narrative, comes to know himself only after immense suffering, and the act of recognizing himself corresponds to the tragic realization of the impossibility of his love, because it lacks the dimension of the other:

> It is myself, I well perceive! It is mine image sure
> That, in this sort deluding me, this fury doth procure!
> I am enamoured of myself; I do both set on fire
> And am the same that swelteth too through impotent desire.
> What shall I do? Be wooed or woo? Whom shall I woo therefore?
> The thing I seek is in myself; my plenty makes me poor.
> O would to God I for a while might from my body part!
> This wish is strange to hear – a lover wrappèd all in smart
> To wish away the thing the which he loveth as his heart!
> My sorrow takes away my strength. I have not long to live
> But in the flower of youth must die. To die it doth not grieve,
> For that by death shall come the end of all my grief and pain.
> I would this youngling whom I love might lenger life obtain,
> For in one soul shall now decay we steadfast lovers twain.[1]

Leiriope, Narcissus's mother, had consulted Teiresias about her son's future, to find out if he would have a long life and reach old age; the blind prophet replied that he would do so if he did not learn to know himself. It is self-knowledge, then, that leads Narcissus to his death, while at the same time offering him the chance of a new life. For Narcissus dies with respect to his complex and turns into 'a flower with a crocus-coloured heart surrounded by white petals', a symbol of rebirth to the unostentatious simplicity of the things of life.

Every transformation in the *Metamorphoses* is the result of a tension of opposites which generates a passion so intense as to induce a change into a new state, a new beginning – in our example, the blooming of the flower Narcissus. Egoic inflation leads to the necessary deflation which, if translated into greater awareness, carries with it the seeds of a new beginning, an ego enriched with both emotional and cognitive significance. At the crucial moment of conflict, one has an intuition of the 'other', of the encounter with difference as an authentic life-moment given to the self. The experience of the conflict generates the possibility of this intuition, a melancholy one because the experience of the 'inner evil' and the tension of its containment is profoundly tragic, especially for the narcissist. However, it is also the necessary condition for being able to smile about oneself, integrating ambivalences and putting an end to collusiveness with the destructive: for as Jung said, the shadow, if we do not know it, if we do not place it in front of ourselves as something different from ourselves, becomes charged with libidinal intensity until it catches the ego by surprise and overrides the conscious address,[2] causing unconscious invasions and types of behaviour that are harmful to ourselves and to others. On the emotional level, this is equivalent to withdrawing the projection of our own shadow on to the other, which is the aspect of ourselves that we do not like, or that we would not like to be or like others to be. This leads us to understand the harmfulness for the psyche of the invention of an external enemy, of the other as an ontological alternative. The original complex does not change, but because it is recognized, its emotional charge is contained and becomes a source of usable energy, no longer imprisoned or opposed; the repetition compulsion is revealed and can be interrupted.

The acceptance of the internal dimension of evil humanizes it; in this way guilt, too, becomes acceptable, because it is commensurate with the real and remediable, instead of being denied, repressed or, conversely, amplified until it reaches unreal dimensions. For some people, this entails realizing that there can be something other than the inevitability of loss, and cultivating an inner discipline of the soul that makes this awareness newly relevant every time.

According to Calvino, Ovid's world is made up of the qualities, attributes and forms that characterize the variety of things, whether plants, animals or persons. But these, he argues, are only outward manifestations of a single common substance which, if stirred by profound emotion, may be transformed into something quite different.[3]

This passage from the first of Calvino's *Memos for the Next Millennium*, 'Lightness', has an analogous relationship with the dynamic of opposites, which plays a central role in analytical psychology. The 'metamorphosis' represents the risk of the dissolution of the personality when the extreme tension between pairs of opposites belonging to the sphere of the collective unconscious is interiorized. The assimilation of such unconscious content into the inventory of individual psychic functions carries a high risk of a dissolution of the ego.[4] When we, as individuals, are unable to differentiate from ourselves the content of the unconscious and access it directly, we may undergo an inundation of meaning, which destroys the thin boundaries of consciousness, and thus erases our identity. Narcissus's speech, which is quoted above, is the tragic and symbolic expression of finally having become aware, at both a rational and an emotional level, of that pole of opposites that is the origin of self-perception, which counterposes the 'me' to the 'non me', thus unveiling a catastrophic truth because it reveals to him the impossibility of a foundation for his identity.

The loss of the sense of limit

In narcissism, a lack of maternal care (expressed in the myth by the violent way in which Narcissus is conceived, Leiriope being raped by Cephissus) causes a weakening of this primary sense of the identity. So all that remains is a desperate and unconscious attempt at compensation, through a constant search for the other in our own reflected image. The reality of the other, in the sense of a desiring difference, a possibility of reciprocal recognition, cannot be perceived and remains indifferent, unless it reflects, or rather 'echoes', a semblance of the self; the other supplies the construction of the self as artifice. Narcissus cannot do without this continual amplification, necessarily transitory and therefore cyclically self-renewing, which translates into a prevalence of role identification (the *per-sona* – literally something that 'sounds through' – was originally the mask of the Roman theatre and later came to denote the set of modalities that each person shows to the world).[5] This search for the mirror of the other – or rather, for the other as mirror – will continue indefinitely, for it cannot be assuaged by the temporary possession of external attributes, of success or fame. It will remain fixed to childhood emotional deprivation and self-pity, to the envy that can accept nothing but the possibility of the absolute enjoyment of the object, in which the other serves only as the mirror on the wall that reflects our own longings.

This condition is expressed in the myth of Echo, whose love is 'heard' by Narcissus only because she repeats *his own* words, but *he rejects* the contact and the relationship, because he finds them unimaginable and therefore unbearable. Echo's devotion, however, is matched by the inner emotional void by which Narcissus is in fact tormented but of which he is completely unaware. In embracing him, only to be violently pushed away, Echo forces him to be aware of his own body, if only for an instant. He is not indifferent to the nymph; quite the contrary – her interest is essential to him as a precondition for living, because it represents the only possible link with otherness, but in the constantly negative mode of rejection. Unnurtured by love, this link grows thinner, like the body in anorexia, eventually disappearing and becoming mere repetitive sound. The denial of the body, of instinctual life, and the inability to feel are a corollary of the whole structure of the myth and of the related complex.

The myth of Narcissus is of particular importance with regard to medicine for two reasons: in the first place, as has already been mentioned, because of the spread of pathological narcissism in contemporary society; in the second place, because of the role it plays in the loss of a sense of moral responsibility and the falsification of culture in our society. Today the search for assuagement is becoming endless, with the incessant roaming of a collective narcissistic spectre which avoids or does not feel its own suffering and is devoid, without necessarily knowing it, of the dimension of the other. A spectre, as in the line of poetry quoted earlier, which never dies to itself, while it is reflected (and wounded, though not mortally) in the countless mirrors that surround it.

The fact of stopping at the literal value, or materializing into objects the images that float to the surface of the mind from the deep sea of inner representations, derives from a limited ability to give value to the possible metaphorical meaning, to make conscious the dimension of inner imaginings which imprints its uniqueness on one's experience of the world. This feeling and understanding of one's own images provides human beings with a position in the world and satisfies their nature at the same time.

When this does not happen, the human being's becoming can translate into a drift of consciousness, and the desire to live can become impossible to assuage. The loss of a sense of the limitedness of human existence generates a continual bulimia for concrete objects – for anything that the human being's natural appetite may identify, on each individual occasion, as an object of their desire.

In present-day society, Narcissism is 'embodied' in the collective consciousness, de-subjectivized but also de-pathologized, and becomes related to socio-economic expectations. In this context, it is legitimate to ask whether an ethical dimension is still possible. It seems unlikely that it could derive from a process of collective self-regulation, while the individual's abstraction from the dimension of the other is normalized, making the process difficult even at an individual level. Today, as Umberto Galimberti points out, Nietzsche's exhortation, *'Werde, wer du bist!'*, 'Become who you are!', is obstructed, if not rendered impossible. In a widely narcissistic context, human beings have great difficulty in knowing the limitations (according to the measure, κατὰ μέτρον, *kata metron*) of their virtue (ἀρετή, *arete*), for they do not accept it, because it is mortal. Hence the philosopher's frequent exhortation to young people to know their own virtue and make it flourish, to set their own *daimon* free, to be in contact with their own talent and cultivate it, facing up to the effort that this entails.[6]

In the media's constant flouting of limitations and morality, the risk remains that of absorbing pre-established external models, which are still the fluctuating *prêt-a-porter* ones of the consumer society.

Examples of omnipotent solitude

A common feature is the one-sided extroversion of our societies: in order to avoid looking inside ourselves, living with negative emotions or facing up to the complexities of the inner world, we prefer to stop at the surface and search there for constant anchorage, firm ground on which to act. But without any internal processing, we end up projecting on to others our own negative emotions, the hidden, denied or repressed inner world. And even if in this case our acts acquire a particularly attractive aura, because we ourselves will continue to entertain the illusion that we are in control of our own house, until we are contradicted, sometimes violently, by the consequences of our acts, by other people's reactions and/or by a sense of having lost our integrity. In this way, the decisions, choices and modes of behaviour 'lose the name of action'.

The collective culture of doing, of taking responsibility for the complexities and to some extent of the basic necessities of most people, helps us to avoid the burden of choice. But this comes at a price – that of making ourselves less free. This reduced freedom is the final outcome of our culture of technological efficiency. In order to meet the financial needs of growth, the narcissistic/hedonistic culture gave a strong impulse to the consumer society, especially at the end of the economic boom, after the 1970s, when the affluence that had been achieved had brought growth to a level of relative stability. Starting in those years, growth reached a saturation point in western societies, and capitalism, becoming global, systematically promoted an individualistic culture, which ideologically gives primacy to the interests of the individual and holds that an extreme individualism is the necessary condition for any 'natural' equilibrium of human society, for the homoeostasis of the global system. Implicit in this conviction is the promise of a further increase in affluence, freedom and social equality, but what actually happened was the exact opposite.

The economic gap, the difference in earnings, with the progressive erosion of the middle class and the welfare state, has never grown as fast as it is growing today. The logic of de-regulation, privatization and the delocalization of work have been its economic corollaries. But the postmodern world continues to promote the external and functional myth of bourgeois affluence, systematically boosting the 'external *locus*' and depathologizing Narcissism.

There are well-adapted people with an unimpaired ability for initiative who continue to function well in society, increasingly striking roots not in their feelings, but in the pragmatic planning energy of rationality, in the overall vision oriented towards the result. They often rise to leading positions, drawing on resources that come from a purely Apollonian dimension. Excelling in distinctive reason, but not integrating their feelings, in fact being able to split them, they are at their ease in the elevated but cold world of ideas and projects, in the sphere of abstract or productive rationality, which defines and decides everything through science and technology. Understanding requires completeness, fullness of language (including the emotional sphere), awareness of the other, and an ability to explore one's own soul to discover the value of things. Sensitivity here loses the implication of connection, compassion, nearness; freedom in affective exchange, in mutual recognition, the basis of all relationships, seems to have been lost. The distance between the two levels seems unbridgeable, while an emotional poverty, a lack of articulation, undermines the spiritual and ethical aspect of social institutions. One could delineate general profiles of libidinal behaviour, active centres of force in society, which strongly condition the way it functions. The patriarchal 'Apollonian' planning character identifies with science and technology, with the practising professions in the various fields of knowledge. But this functionality based on specialization is matched by a 'splitting of the libidinal dimension'. The eros, strongly exposed to exploitation by the market, loses its peculiarly spiritual qualities, and ignores the broader and more refined dimension of the body and pleasure.

Another example of narcissistic omnipotence is the so-called 'social networks', notably Facebook, which is widely used in hospitals, as elsewhere. The Internet is the place of circulation of the content of the collective unconscious, whose images are projected on to the virtual screen of the net. Wolfgang Giegerich puts it as follows:

> The place of real life, of where the heart of society beats, the place of 'the soul', is out there 'behind' the screen, in the Web, no longer in

us. In ourselves we only find the subjective soul, our personal feelings and fantasies, not what Jung termed the 'objective', 'transpersonal', or 'autonomous' psyche (which he, however, still tried to locate in the individual). The Web is truly transpersonal, largely independent of the individual.[7]

In the social networks, projection is strongly stimulated as the prevalent psychological mode. The medium becomes an anonymous and impersonal container. The natural variety of the possibilities of a relationship with the real person, consisting of a direct confrontation with the thoughts, intuitions, feelings, sensations, variably expressed in the spontaneous richness of language, is reduced and changed. The need for company, for avoiding solitude, is amplified, and the search for immediacy of stimulus can become compulsive, in much the same way as was described above with regard to inverse initiation in consumerism. The virtual image of the other represents an elsewhere, an imaginary place and time, invested with projections. This mode of libidinal investment in the Web may satisfy the immediate need for the other, but it does not meet a neutral medium. Individuals cannot be represented in their entirety or in their mystery. The risk is that the recipients are spectators of a dreaming, self-referential tendency, which can include moments of authentic confrontation only within very restricted limits.

The images' power of fascination may coercively induce a predominance of virtual psychic space over reality, even when one knows the person at the other point in the Web. The sense of distance becomes ingrained and acquires pre-eminence over the real proximity of the other.

The unconscious nostalgia for an aesthetic, mythical container, replaced by the 'virtual' world of the Web, always ready for consumption and interchangeable, seems to manifest itself in this parallel space. A form of re-enchantment, oriented by the market, which replaces nature with the electronic prostheses of the ego and creates around each person an artificial environment in their own image and likeness. In hospitals, too, and not only outside working hours, relationships are interwoven in the parallel space for the projection of one's desire for signification and meeting, a surrogate for the spaces of creativity that the world of work frequently does not offer.

A more widespread form of behaviour is that of not explaining to patients, not giving them the information that they need, adapting one's discourse to their capacity for taking things in and understanding them. The reason, once again, is the doctor's inability to stop and listen. To listen patiently and observe constantly, creating the space of a dialogue with the man or woman in front of you, putting yourself openly in front of them, on the same level, waiting in silence for them to finish their sentences, so that they don't feel that they need to fill the silence by rushing. To start from this kind of listening, and choose your words carefully, with simplicity, to explain, interact and offer the patient who so desires a greater possibility of self-determination in choice. More generally, this active openness constitutes the basis for a non-manipulative involvement of the patient in the healing process. A non-reductive approach to communication brings complexity, but also significance, to the process. Unfortunately, it is impeded, if not made impossible, by the tyranny of the time allotted for treatment and by a resistance, of cultural origin, on the part of some patients. Doctors tend to use, in a more or less conscious way, the strong, convincing power of reason and scientific terminology, and think they can eliminate the sphere of subjective communication. The importance of this point should not be underestimated, for on it depends the possibility of moving medicine beyond the mechanical nature of individual 'services' towards a culture, and an economic structure, oriented towards the person. The final result could then emerge from a decision-making process involving both parties, while the reimbursement no longer refers to all the services provided, but becomes dependent on the result achieved in a process that directly involves the patient.

Many years ago, Jung made the following observation on the medical profession:

> The study of medicine consists on the one hand in storing up in the mind an enormous number of facts, which are simply memorized without any real knowledge of their foundations, and on the other hand in learning practical skills, which have to be acquired on the principle 'Don't think, act!' Thus it is that, of all the professionals, the medical man has the least opportunity of developing the function of *thinking*.[8]

Too often doctors are content to become human prostheses of an 'action culture', which through demography and techno-capitalist development has reached proportions unimaginable in Jung's time; it has never been so urgent as it is today to develop the function of thinking in doctors – and by this I mean critical thinking, not thinking exclusively applied to empirical action – in the context of a profession which is breaking through in such important areas of human life as disease, suffering and death.

As an example of omnipotence on the part of the patient, I am reminded of a man close to retirement age, a shop owner, who would always become particularly obsessed with work in the period leading up to Christmas. For two months he had been hiding from himself and from his family the progressive symptoms of angina pectoris. His denial had reached such a point that he refused to go to casualty even when he had a particularly prolonged attack of angina on Christmas Day itself. A few days later he had to be rushed to the nearest hospital suffering from severe breathing difficulties and pains in his chest. He had had a pulmonary oedema, which causes a feeling sometimes likened to 'drowning inside yourself'. The diagnosis also revealed that he had had a heart attack, probably on Christmas Day. This had led to his present symptoms of heart failure, which had grown progressively over the following days. The illness was a terrible blow to him, because he lacked the courage that might have been provided by closeness to himself and to his family. Even after being taken to hospital, once he had got over his initial dismay, he somehow denied the reality of what had happened to him, not trusting the judgement of the doctors in the 'small' hospital where he had been taken. He would say, 'Nothing serious happened to me at all. It was the doctors in the other hospital who said I'd had a heart attack. In fact I was fine, I never had anything of the kind. It was just a passing thing.' Refusing to undergo further treatment, he requested a transfer to the 'bigger' university hospital nearby. Here, convinced that he could eliminate the remotest possibility of any problem, he thought he would meet the personification of modern *auctoritas*, the impersonal goddess of Science: 'You people really are good, in fact you're excellent. You've completely cured me with your incredible skills!' In this way he could avoid his terror and accept his illness, but only through this optimistic and impersonal projection on to the new doctors, true avatars of a superior knowledge that can solve every problem. He was still unaware of his anxiety and fear, and of the related pressure. The grandiosity of his projection on to rational empirical medicine and on to the principle of causality, though it made him experience the illness as a nightmare, was the only thing that could counterbalance the abyss of his sense of loss, connected with the bodily revelation of his vulnerability. Because of the seriousness of his initial denial, only the implicit promise of a nobler therapeutic redemption, of first-class treatment, could protect him from having to accept the experience of illness as a vehicle of meaning, but hopefully also give him another possibility of processing it.

Epilogue: the weight of limit and unlimited hope

The example just described illustrates the sense of limit as an ability to see reality for what it is, and therefore to feel and see one's own body and its signals. The chorus of *Oedipus at Colonus* says:

> Whoso craves the ampler length of life, not content to desire a modest span, him will I judge with no uncertain voice; he cleaves to folly. For the long days lay up full many things nearer unto grief than joy; but as for thy delights, their place shall know them no more, when a man's life hath lapsed beyond the fitting term.[9]

Today, unlike in the days when the tragedy was written, since priority is given to the theme of individual responsibility, the withdrawal of projections has become fundamental, as a presupposition of any authentic ethical position.[10] Paying attention to the unconscious makes it possible for us to know the shadow and to withdraw the projections. The sense of tragedy consists in recognizing that the evil is also internal, that it is a potentiality that concerns everyone (something which today may seem obvious); this may make us anxious and sad, because we realize that we are vulnerable, but at the same time it confronts us with the burden of the limitedness of our existence as interconnected individuals and as mortals. 'You cannot even distinguish the pleasant things' if you cross the boundary; if you do not make the effort to recognize it, you will not be able to recognize your virtue and exercise power in your life; this enables you, insofar as it is within your power, not to waste it. As Nietzsche points out, from the point of view of the classical pessimism of the Greeks, to recognize the naturalness of limitation – that is, of death – does not mean developing a depressive relationship with existence; on the contrary, it is an incentive to live life to the full, an affirmation of the whole of life, a saying yes to this life even in the sense of its power (however limited that power may be). This leads to the recognition that the great joy of living is also accompanied by great sorrow, and to the possibility of empathy.[11] Nietzsche counters classical pessimism with the nihilism of resignation to the nothingness of existence, whereby the only authentic life is that after death.[12] In contrast, romantic pessimism, which sentimentalizes the tragic, losing sight of the conflict inherent in the nature of things, represented, as it still does today, a highway for the philosophies of consolation, including the New Age, in contemporary society.

In Christian monotheism, absolute hope links life with the certainty of redemption, and this makes any sorrow bearable. Sorrow is justified by sin and guilt; it is not an original condition. The necessary overcoming of sorrow testifies to the pact of alliance, election and elevation in the history of

God's people, which always looks forward to a new period of waiting for the Saviour's coming, which is absolutely certain, but always placed in an indefinable future time. In medicine, suffering becomes assimilable to atonement; death is considered illusory.

Tragedy, hidden in the proximity between life and power, power and death, death and regeneration, is the tension between the contrasting needs of the individual, whose death is the inevitable end of a single unrepeatable whole, and of *physis*, the being or nature that comprises all forms of life. For *physis*, death is necessary to the regeneration of new life – that is, to the happiness of everything. The energy and joy of renewal is inseparable from the cruelty of the deaths of the individual entities that constitute being. When individuals risk their lives, relishing the joy of living, they discover the inevitability of sorrow and the proximity of death. The tension of closeness to the boundary, which is also knowledge of the threshold of inflation, is revealed to be a necessity. Hence the ambiguity of every action, which draws a thin, sensitive line in the consciousness, stretched taut between the effort of carrying the weight of limitation on the one hand and the exercise of power on the other.

This paradoxical tension of life makes Dionysus – the god who was torn limb from limb – the one closest to the meaning of tragedy. After he is killed by the Titans (Prometheus's brothers) his heart will be preserved and later brought back to life by his father Zeus. Kerényi states in the *Gods of the Greeks* that those two Titans were considered the precursors of humankind.[13] Dionysus represents the state of nature, generative but also a primal, savage, instinctual frenzy, a mixture of cruelty and happiness, a euphoria that overflows with life but kills. Dionysus is not harmonious and symmetrical, corresponding to principles of scientific or aesthetic harmony, like Apollo. In a manner analogous to Asclepius, he must be considered the god who is closest to human mortality, because he was born from a dying mother, because he was killed by the Titans and because he travelled down into the Underworld in search of his mother Semele. Significantly, in another version of the myth he is born to Zeus and Persephone, the 'queen of Hades' (or of death). Mortal hope, the dismemberment of Dionysus, and the metaphysics of the tragic are replaced by the eschatological certainty of Christ's suffering on the cross, through which salvation has already been guaranteed.[14] This principle of absolute hope will be handed down to medicine too, and will acquire the means for responding to the expectations of treatment, to accomplish – hoping against hope – even that which is seemingly impossible, bringing to linguistic expression and inserting into history the fundamental hopes of all human beings.

It is worth noting, in this connection, that since the community and technology replaced nature and the individual in the exercise of power, there has been a reduction of biodiversity and of diversity in general. This is indicative of how the unconsciousness of nature, the predominance of its 'pleasure principle', which combines cruelty and happiness, was essential to the manifold differentiation of life forms. In the contemporary age, however, the prevailing attitude is a technological view of the world as uniformity and quantity. This view is channelled into medical treatment, through the unreflecting automatisms and collective conformities of protocols. While the diversity of animal and plant life diminishes, it is clear that human pleasure, in its narcissistic sense, once it is made global, is perhaps more uniform, and therefore controllable (easier to integrate in the Web society), but unsustainable, and therefore highly damaging to the species as a whole. Moreover, the limits of the expansion of the species are also becoming clear, because urbanization is associated with a progressive reduction in human fertility. However, these signals have not yet reached such a level of significance as to compel humanity to opt for greater intergenerational solidarity and a greater respect for nature.

Notes

1 Ovid, p. 110 (Book III, lines 463–473, in the Latin text).
2 Jung 1953, p. 73.
3 Calvino 1988, p. 9.
4 See Jung 1953, p. 149: 'If through assimilation of the unconscious we make the mistake of including the collective psyche in the inventory of personal psychic functions, a dissolution of the personality into its paired opposites inevitably follows.'
5 Jung 1959, pp. 122–123:

> A common instance of this is identity with the persona, which is the individual's system of adaptation to, or the manner he assumes in dealing with, the world. Every calling or profession has its own characteristic persona. [. . .] Only, the danger is that they become identical with their personas – the professor with his textbook, the tenor with his voice. [. . .] One could say, with a little exaggeration, that the persona is that which in reality one is not, but which oneself as well as others think one is. In any case the temptation to be what one seems to be is great, because the persona is usually rewarded in cash.

6 Galimberti 2008.
7 Giegerich 2007, p. 314.
8 Jung 1960, p. 277.
9 Sophocles, pp. 104–105.
10 Neumann 1948.
11 The two attitudes described above coincide with the distinctive characters of the paranoid-schyzoid and depressive positions in psychoanalytical literature.
12 Nietzsche 1887–88, pp. 12–14.
13 *Orphic Hymn*, 37.2, cit. in Kerényi 1951, p. 255. The resurrection of the slain god, in ancient Egypt, had already been described in the myth of Osiris, the precursor of the myth of Dionysus Zagreus, to the point where they were identified

with each other in Greco-Roman cities of the first centuries A.D., such as Anti-noopolis or Philadelphia, in an era and in places that saw the births of Apuleius, Plotinus and later Augustine (see Doxiadis 1995, p. 46). A fundamental differ-ence between the two myths is that the dismembering of Osiris, in the Egyptian myth, is the work of Set, a symbol of the shadow in its archetypal 'classical' sense (the shadow as primal envy, thirsty for non-legitimate power, pure destructive-ness), who is later revealed to be a paradoxical stimulus to the rebirth and dif-ferentiation of the consciousness – in the form of the sun god, Horus.

14 Natoli 1986, p. 203.

Bibliography

Calvino, Italo (1988), *Lezioni Americane: Sei Proposte per il Prossimo Millennio. Six Memos for the Next Millennium: The Charles Eliot Norton Lectures 1985–86*, translated by Patrick Creagh, London: Penguin Modern Classics, 1993.

Doxiadis, Euphrosyne (1995), *The Mysterious Fayum Portraits: Faces from Ancient Egypt*, London: Thames & Hudson, 1995.

Galimberti, Umberto (2008), *L'ospite Inquietante*, Milan: Feltrinelli, 2008.

Giegerich, Wolfgang (2007), *Technology and the Soul: From the Nuclear Bomb to the World Wide Web*, Collected English Papers, Vol. 2, New Orleans, LA: Spring Journal Books, 2007.

Jung, Carl Gustav (1953), *Zwei Schriften über Analytische Psychologie. Two Essays on Analytical Psychology*, Bollingen Series XX, Vol. 7 of the Collected Works of C.G. Jung, translated by Richard Francis Carrington Hull, London & New York: Rout-ledge, 1990.

Jung, Carl Gustav (1959), *Die Archetypen und das Kollektive Unbewußte. The Archetypes and the Collective Unconscious*, Bollingen Series XX, Vol. 9, Part I of the Collected Works of C.G. Jung, translated by Richard Francis Carrington Hull, Princeton, NJ: Princeton University Press, 1969.

Jung, Carl Gustav (1960), *Die Dynamik des Unbewußten. The Structure and Dynam-ics of the Psyche*, Bollingen Series XX, Vol. 8 of the Collected Works of C.G. Jung, translated by Richard Francis Carrington Hull, Princeton, NJ: Princeton University Press, 1969.

Kerényi, Karl (1951), *Die Mythologie der Griechen. The Gods of the Greeks*, Lon-don: Thames & Hudson, 2008.

Klein, Melanie (1946), 'Notes on Some Schizoid Mechanisms', in *The Selected Mela-nie Klein*, Juliet Mitchell, London: Penguin Books, 1986.

Natoli, Salvatore (1986), *L'Esperienza del Dolore: Le Forme del Patire nella Cultura Occidentale. The Experience of Pain: The Forms of Suffering in Western Culture*, Milan: Feltrinelli, 2008.

Neumann, Erich (1948), *Tiefenspychologie und Neue Ethik. Depth Psychology and a New Ethic*, translated by Eugene Rolfe, Boston & London: Shambala, 1990.

Nietzsche, Friedrich (1887–88), *Frammenti Postumi, 1887–1888. Posthumous Frag-ments, 1997–1888*, translated by Sossio Giametta, Milan: Adelphi, 1971.

Ovid, *Metamorphoses*, translated by Arthur Golding, edited by Madeleine Forey, London: Penguin Books, 2002.

Sophocles, *The Tragedies*, translated into English prose by Sir Richard C. Jebb, Cam-bridge: Cambridge University Press, 1904.

Chapter 5

The illusory nature of concretism

The inner spectator, the harpsichord

By the reality of the psyche, Donald Kalsched means 'an intermediate realm of experience, which serves as a ligament connecting the inner self and the outer world by means of symbolic processes which communicate a sense of "meaning".'[1]

In Greek mythology the twin giants Otus and Ephialtes were known as the Aloadae. According to Homer's description, they were very handsome and grew a stade[2] higher and a cubit wider every year. Like the giants in the Gigantomachia, the Aloadae dared to challenge the gods. When they were still small, they imprisoned Ares, the god of war, in a bronze vessel, where he remained for thirteen months, until Hermes set him free. At the age of nine, even bolder, they decided to climb up into the heavens by putting Mount Pelion on top of Mount Ossa, to reach a height equal to that of Mount Olympus. The Aloadae feared no one, for it had been foretold that they would never be killed, either by human beings or by gods. Ephialtes wanted to rape Hera, and Otus had the same designs on Artemis. Artemis went to meet them, in the form of a doe. The two giants, vying with each other in their skill as hunters, each threw a javelin at the animal from opposite sides. The goddess in the form of a doe deftly dodged the weapons, but the two brothers were unable to do the same, and killed each other. Artemis in animal form is here a metaphor for the concretism and superior vision of the gods, who are able to anticipate the literal vision of the giants, who would not understand the deception because they were unable to transcend appearances. Blind to the metaphorical meaning of reality and driven by the desire to outdo each other, they achieve the only possible result, their own deaths.

Jorge Luis Borges, in a lecture he gave in 1966 on Samuel Johnson, as seen by his official biographer, Boswell,[3] made a comment on the latter's experience. According to a pre-fifth-century Hindu school of thought, he said, we are all spectators of our lives rather than actors in them, like an audience watching a dancer. The same is true today. We see an actor or dancer playing a part on the stage, or read about a character in a novel, and we identify with them. The same happens in real life. He himself, he remarked, had been born on the same day as Jorge Luis Borges; throughout his life he had watched him act admirably on some occasions, less nobly on others, and he had come to identify with him, while always aware of being a separate entity. Borges described this experience as that of a 'double I', comprising on the one hand a profound I and on the other a separate I who, especially at times when something very good or bad happened to him, felt as if it were happening to someone else. He compares this experience to that of the character Parolles in Shakespeare's *All's Well That Ends Well*, who at first convinces everyone that he was a war hero, and is rewarded with medals and promotion. When he is found out, he is stripped of his medals and publicly shamed; but nevertheless he resolves that, though no longer a captain, he will live on as himself. 'He says "simply the thing I am shall make me live" . . . within us'. That is, he feels that above and beyond the circumstances, beyond his cowardice, his humiliation, he is something else, a kind of strength we all have within us.' That something within the self, comparable to Spinoza's 'God', Schopenhauer's 'will', Bernard Shaw's 'life force' and Bergson's 'vital impulse', would survive the humiliation and the loss. Borges held that this was precisely what Boswell had gone through.

In a session of analysis a patient once told me how, when he was a boy, while listening to the first movement, the Largo, of Bach's Fifth Violin Sonata, he had had an intuition, a flash of inspiration, which would later serve him as a guide in many situations of his life. He thought that the two main voices of the piece represented two different modes of his existence. The first was expressed by the violin, with its melodic tendency, its leaps and bounds, and its variations, now lyrical, now melancholic. This first, more linear voice expressed his participation in the things of the world, in its varying fortunes, the courage to take risks in life and dive into its sea, but also the rational leaps of the mind, the challenges of knowledge. The second voice, the harpsichord, incessantly repeated a circular melodic scheme, with slight variations of tone and colour, so delicate as to be barely perceptible, but in constant dialogue with the soaring leaps of the violin. Only at certain crucial points, of greater lyrical intensity, did the basic constancy and rhythmicality of the second voice tend to quicken its pace, but this would last only for a short parenthesis, in accordance with the needs of metre and harmony. This cyclical inner voice seemed to him to form a constant background to experience, like a more essential, deeper timbre of the continuity of life. The tension of the interplay between the two voices, in their reciprocal effort to harmonize in dialogue with one another, while maintaining two different rhythms, reminded the listener of his responsibility to take hold of his own passion, his own desire, and of the discipline of continual interaction and self-questioning in relation with the other, to which the harmony refers as a whole. For in his experience, if one does not listen to both voices, an effort which requires constant discipline, one is at greater risk of losing the inter-subjective dimension of desire, and respect for its mystery; one can fall into the illusion of concretism, or into the temptation of the absolute object and its consumption.

The inner imbalance between the two voices can lead the violin's voice, no longer restrained by the circular rhythm of the harpsichord, to tip the balance, usually towards the outside. That can lead one to betray the command of desire, to remove the requirement of limitation, interiorizing the hedonistic message of the times, the infinite dimension of enjoyment of a 'disposable', Don Giovanni-like, kind of living.

It takes an active imagination, openness and attention to the images of the unconscious to see how they are related to the external images that are continually presented to the senses by life, by the media machine and by the language of the simulacrum in the post-modern era.

Knowledge by difformity as an antidote to the bulimia of desire: the more we see things through the mirror of absurd animal images, chimerical creatures, enigmatic forms, bizarre personifications of vices and bestial instincts, expressions of the desiring impulses that do not originate in the ego, but reach it and inspire it, the more it is possible to unveil the human being's inner complexity, its truth. This implies that imagination will be less able to be placated by 'carnal', merely concretistic, enjoyment of the object. The residual alienation will drive it to enter a dimension of openness, making an effort of observation, research and imaginal reflection. This effort is continually confronted by the seduction of the abyss that lies below all enjoyment and, at the same time, by the temptation of a fundamentalist drift towards the demonization of evil.

Before coming to love the beloved, we must therefore recognize the luxury (from *luxus*, dislocation) of the desiring impulses, which are only sated by themselves, through the illusions of concretism, the objects made absolute by the compulsive projection of our unlived lives. Counterposed to happiness, and to the right to seek it, as the enjoyment of consumption indefinitely reproduced as an end in itself, is '*eudaimonia*', serenity as a process for those who take the trouble to confront their own inner demon and the necessary illusions of desire.

By contrast, the mysticism of Rumi (1207–1273), the great Persian Sufi poet of the thirteenth century, founder of the Order of Dervishes (in Konya, Turkey), refers to the mirror of the heart as a rough metal which distorts the images of objects, and whose surface must therefore be smoothed by spiritual discipline, becoming so pure that it can reflect the beloved's true face, but without divulging it to everyone, keeping it secret inside itself.

> Dismiss cares and be utterly clear of heart,
> Like the face of a mirror without image and picture.
> When it becomes clear of images, all images are contained in it;
> No man's face is ashamed of that clear-faced one.
> Wouldst thou have a clear mirror, behold thyself therein.
> For it is not ashamed or afraid of telling the truth.
> Since the steel face gained this purity by discrimination,
> What needs the heart's face, which has no dust?
> But betwixt the steel and the heart is this difference,
> That the one is a keeper of secrets, while the other is not.[4]

In an oral tradition of Senegalese Sufism (communicated to me in a private conversation), the ego, as in a metallurgical procedure, is first made incandescent by the fire of God's desire, then hammered, bent and moulded until a form is forged which is his alone. One could take other examples from Dante's *Paradiso*, where the symbolisms of the eye, the heart and the mirror are fused with and superimposed on each other.

In the world of healthcare, the doctors' loss of a 'philosophical' and imaginal attitude towards their everyday choices has led to the *furor agendi* so characteristic of present-day hospitals. Evidence-based medicine often does not consider the second level, that of the inner spectator who listens, records and comments, and probably, if invited to do so, could tell a different story and suggest new thoughts to us.

Notes

1 Kalsched 1996, pp. 6–7.
2 'The name *stadium* derives from the Greek unit of measurement, the *stade*, the distance covered in the original Greek footraces (about 600 feet [180 metres]). The course for the footrace in the ancient Olympic Games at was exactly a stade in length, and the word for the unit of measurement became transferred first to the footrace and then to the place in which the race was run'. From: www.britannica.com/technology/stadium#ref100143 Accessed 5th November 2017.
3 Borges 2013, p. 97. 'A Lecture on Johnson and Boswell', *New York Review of Books*, July 28, 2013, Excerpted from '*Class 10: Samuel Johnson as Seen by Boswell. The Art of Biography. Johnson and His Critics*. Monday, November 7, 1966,' in *Professor Borges: A Course on English Literature*, a compilation of twenty-five lectures Borges gave in 1966. www.nybooks.com/daily/2013/07/28/lecture-johnson-and-boswell Accessed 30th October 2017.
4 Jalāl al-Dīn Rūmī 1898, p. 53.

Bibliography

Borges, Jorge Luis (2013), *Professor Borges: A Course on English Literature*, translated by Katherine Silver, New York: New Directions, 2013.

Jalāl al-Dīn Rūmī, Maulana, *Selected Poems from the Dīvāni Shamsi Tabrīz*, edited and translated with an introduction, notes and appendices by Reynold A. Nicholson, Cambridge: Cambridge University Press, 1898.

Kalsched, Donald (1996), *The Inner World of Trauma: Archetypal Defences of the Personal Spirit*, London: Routledge, 1996.

Chapter 6

Considerations on courage

Courage in our time

The common etymological root of the words 'courage' – from Vulgar Latin *coraticum*, ultimately from Latin *cor* (the heart) – and 'record', but also 'crown', seems to recall the intimate link between time, memory and essence, between the heart as the centre of being and the sense of regality. There is a curious parallel with the cardiac anatomy: the 'coronaries' surround the heart as the crown encircles a king or queen's head. The heart is the inner sovereign, the seminal principle of being, the living reality of being and its transformation into continual cycles of life, death and rebirth (systole and diastole). Since time immemorial, in alchemy and astrology, the heart has been associated with such symbols as gold, the sun (outside the cave) – and the lion, an expression of the 'volitional' will of the human being.

But is courage the hero's prerogative? What is there in common between the classical concept of the hero, whose deeds embody the tension of courage, and that of the modern hero, like Camus's Sisyphus, whose courage consists in accepting his own meaningless condition:

> in a universe that is suddenly bereft of illusions and enlightenment, the human being feels like a stranger. There is no remedy for this exile, for it lacks any memories of a lost home country or hope of a promised land.

What implication for courage was there in 'this divorce between the individual and life, between the performer and the stage', which 'is truly the sense of absurdity'?[1]

In a world which is one-sidedly supported by extroversion, and whose reality principle is chiefly that of objectifying representation, it is hard to think of courage as part of a further expansion of rational consciousness, new conquests in the name of reason, or a profound colonization of psychic space. That kind of courage belongs to the history of the last few centuries, but today one senses symptoms of satiety and nausea with it. The concretism

predominant in the era of technology seems to view technological realization, the man of 'action', as the symbol of contemporary courage and heroism. I intend to argue, by contrast, that, in this age of the greatest expansion
of humankind's rational power and of the manipulation of nature, which
has been reduced to an object, another kind of courage can perform an
authentic compensatory action with regard to the spirit of the times: the
courage to renounce one-sidedness, to accept the mission and the enterprise
of embracing the limitedness and totality of our own nature.

> All feelings that encapsulate your essence and uplift it are pure; a feeling
> that expresses only *one* side of your nature and therefore distorts you is
> impure. [. . .] Any heightening is good, if it is in your *whole* blood, if it is
> not intoxication, not smokiness, but joy that can be seen in concrete form.[2]

Rilke, in one of his *Letters to a Young Poet*, represents courage as an inner
act, made up of waiting, doubt and suffering. Its time is one of patient toler-
ance of tension which does not yield to effusions: the patience to experience
questions, to keep to the difficult, not seeking an easy answer, but waiting
for life itself to be completed in an answer which is often not intelligible,
except in hindsight. This expresses the circularity of psychic time, in contrast to the axial linearity of reason. In this symbolic tension, individuation
is revealed as the red line that combines the thousand possible lives of each
one of us in a single narrative.

Only if it is educated to the limit can doubt lose its negative, nihilistic
meaning, and become knowledge, turn into criticism.

> Ask it, whenever it tries to spoil something for you, *why* the thing in ques-
> tion is undesirable; demand that it give you evidence; press it, and you may
> find it to be at a loss for words, embarrassed, maybe even irritable. But
> don't let up; demand proof, respond in the same way every time, showing
> yourself to be punctilious and unrelenting, and the day will come when
> what was once a wrecker turns into one of your finest workers – perhaps
> the most skilled of all those engaged in the project of building your life.[3]

How can we speak of courage without mentioning tales of courageous
men? Hector's gesture remains probably the purest symbol of courage in
historical time. Unlike Achilles, whose overbearing courage will meet its
limit in grief, but also unlike Ulysses, the precursor of modernity in his rationalism already contaminated with utilitarianism, Achilles and Ulysses shed
indecorous tears for themselves if suddenly confronted with emotions they

usually manage to repress: 'Hector possesses a level of congruity which is new for an ancient hero: he has the courage not only to face up to battle, but can also face up to memories and feelings.'[4]

> Hector is different. He again, to be sure, is no stranger to temptation, but not to the temptations of ire, like those which enslave Achilles, nor to those of novelty, which seduce Ulysses. He is tempted by the warmth and reasonability of women. The enticements to which he's exposed are in no way scandalous, and indeed are proffered in a spirit that considers the needs of all. They run counter, however, to the world of his duties. Hector listens to the voices of affection and to proposals that counsel compromise. He understands their motivations and acknowledges their reasonability. And he rejects them for reasons which are free of moral prejudice.[5]

He fights against his own heart (*thymos* or *kardia*) and enriches it with his conscious choice. To be able to embrace his son, he must remove the 'armour', the heart's defensive crust, agreeing to reveal his own nature, so as to feel the child inside him. The gesture, unthinkable for those times, was that of lifting his son above himself, praying to the gods to make him become much stronger than his father. Hector goes into battle consciously, knowing he is going to die in order to carry out the duty dictated to him by his code of honour and a sense of responsibility towards the *polis*. He will die by the hand of the violent competitive male, Achilles, who has rejected fatherhood in exchange for glory. Hector is courageous because he succeeds in facing up to his own inner contradictions, in standing up to the demon of doubt, frequently feeling the temptation of taking the easier route, before carrying the weight of ambivalence and going to meet his destiny.[6]

Today, the armour of the doctor who approaches the patient, often hidden so as not to overemphasize its importance, consists of that normative hypertrophy which insinuates itself into the gap between the market of (specialistic) knowledge and the promise of recovery, between professional corporativism and empathy, made up of 'informed consent' and dissociation between action and emotion. But, as has already been mentioned, the loss of the language of feeling generates moral indistinction, imaginative impotence, the incapacity to face the complexity of the real, and in particular disorientation, if not squalor and desolation, in the inner landscape of the doctor's soul.

If the heart is the seat of that intimate imagination which is the root of the symbolic function, which, keeping the tension between opposites in check, is able to integrate the ambivalences, today it is pervaded by a sense of ineffability and at the same time of absolute solitude. It is unable to dispense with the rational distinctions between subject and object, transcendence and immanence, ego and id, matter and spirit, and is easily imprisoned in the rigid scheme of *tertium non datur*. We have passed from the heart as the unitary seat of being and imagination to the dualism of Harvey's anatomical heart.[7]

As doctors, we can ask ourselves the question: how is it possible for today's doctors to achieve reconciliation with the philosophical spirit of Hippocrates, Galen, Rhazes, Maimonides, Avicenna and Paracelsus? They were philosophers, as well as doctors. How is it possible to develop in our times an opening up of the empirical approach to philosophical examination, in the form of a critical and imaginative spirit which does not restrict itself to a merely functional deployment of the cure, but orients itself towards a parallel cultivation of the soul? Many doctors have also been writers: for example Rabelais, Chekhov, Bulgakov, Céline. There remains a sense of the necessity for all doctors, in their daily practice, to ask themselves this question and look for answers.

St Anthony's Fire

There is also the courage of those who, like St Anthony the Great at the turn of the fourth century AD, abandoned everything and retired to the Egyptian desert, eating nothing but bread and fighting against the temptations of the devil, an eminent example of monastic life, the first conqueror of ascetic space in the inner landscape of Christian monotheism. Asceticism dominates emotions and holds them back, projecting them into a programme, the building of a future, unlimited good. In the country from which Moses escaped, monotheism fled from its archaic origins, across the Red Sea, towards the provident God of reason and of the supreme values that conceal being.

But Anthony is also the saint of the fire that bears that name, the burning evil, its peculiar somatization which expresses the return of the demon of desire, of the temptation to break out of isolation, that superior distance between the self and others, which finds no other way than a 'rash', on the skin, on the somatic interface between the inside and the outside.[8] Anthony, the patron saint of animals, seems to preside over that new relationship with instinctual life (symbolized by animals), which tames the passions of the heart and gives reason priority over instinct. Curiously, a legend of the Veneto region tells how thanks to the saint, here named San Bovo or San Bò, animals gained the faculty of speech on the night of the 17th of January.

Instinct paradoxically takes on the characteristics of the *logos*, the word. For this reason, which is both caricatural and histrionic, but also frightening, the common people kept well away from cattlesheds to avoid the evil eye.

In the history of art, Anthony the abbot is above all the saint of devilish temptations: one immediately thinks of Hieronymus Bosch's triptych (Figure 6.1), where the impulses of the unconscious find the most varied expressions in theriomorphic beings, part human and part beast, which torment the saint as he tries to reach a room inside a ruined building. In the room is a human figure with a halo, the saint worshipping the cross, a metaphor for interiority. All this is going on under the vault of a sky broken up into two sectors: one red with the fire of burning buildings and the other a clear area where caravels sail through the air; the sky is ploughed by a bird-ship, flying fish and winged boats, a possible metaphor for reductive individuation, only possible in a purified celestial space, the expression of a one-sided attitude of the spirit, itself not immune to inflationary, sinful temptations.

There may also be a madness, a fanaticism, a kind of extremism of reason, of logic unmitigated by the moderation of the ego that a mild mysticism brings with it, in people who know they are not the bearers of absolute truths, and feel humbled because their egos do not identify with their limited knowledge. Then there is a completely different asceticism which despises

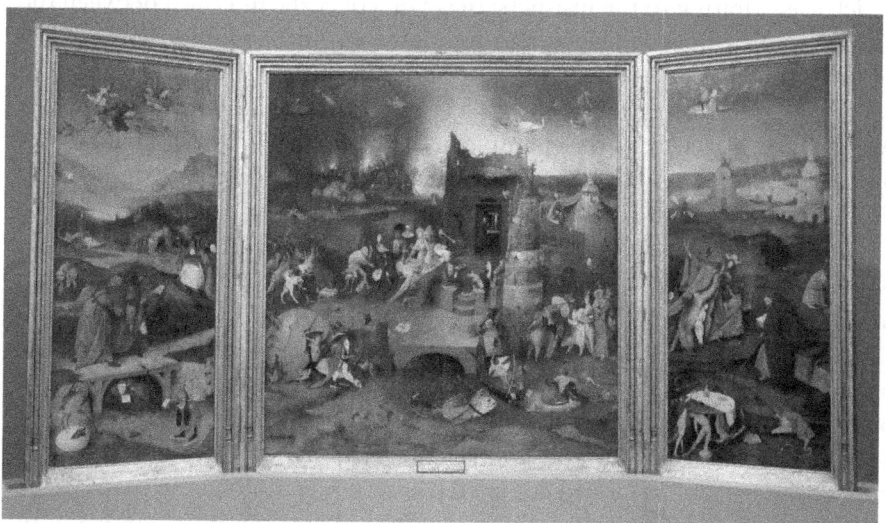

Figure 6.1 Triptych of the Temptation of St Anthony. Hieronymus Bosch. Museu Nacional de Arte Antiga, Lisbon.

the world, projecting its own mystery on to the absolute otherness of a God who transcends not only the ego but the psyche itself, and emanates the collective demands of dogma. If God is projected on to the outside, the self will be unconsciously felt to be a projection. Here too technology remains neutral; indeed it is often used by fundamentalists without any detriment to their literalistic anti-scientific beliefs, such as those that look back on the creation of the world not as a symbol, but as a literal genesis.

The traditional asceticism of the great monotheistic religions is manifested first and foremost in detachment from earthly possessions, from mother earth. Only by losing an aesthetically oriented awe of natural objects can one acquire the detachment necessary for scientific objectivity and the technological manipulation of objects. Only by being objectified can nature be made knowable and manipulable, thus losing its meaning of *mater natura* (just as the word 'matter' loses the maternal sense of its etymological root).

The emancipation of the scientific principle from the magic container of the great mother, the ancient goddess of the Stone Age, finds its greatest propulsive drive in monotheism. Augustine warns human beings to beware of *aesthesis*, love for the things of this world: material possessions, the deceptive beauty of nature, its seas, mountains, rivers, lakes, forests, deserts, boundless skies, starry nights, dawns and sunsets.[9] In the same way it will be possible to observe in the boundary organ all those manifestations which are irritating to the instincts; they will cover the interface between the inner world of human beings and the outer world of mother nature with erythemas, itches or wounds, thus revealing the common embryonic origin of the skin and the nervous system (ectoderm). In the late fourth century, St Augustine was struck by the example of St Anthony, and this contributed to his conversion. In Milan he was baptized in the basilica of St Ambrose by the Saint and Church Father of that name.

Once the aesthetic commandment has been sacrificed, all that remains is the implicitly binary moral commandment of the one God: love nothing but the mystery of God; the aesthetic deception distracts our eyes from the unknowable and ineffable face of God, the only possible true love, the only supreme good. Here a separation is made between the principle of beauty and that of justice, breaking away from the unitary sense of the ancient Greeks' beautiful and good (*kaloskagathos*)[10] towards a scientific knowledge which has moved completely into *physis*, combining mathematical form and technological practice. A sense of the continual epiphany of the divine in the things of the world, of personified nature, of an intimate connection between the human and the divine, is innate in the ancients' soul. Until Augustine, they were completely detached from that sense of the 'ego' as the 'inner' seat of the unfathomable mystery of being. Historically, it is the ascetic face of monotheism that shows the greatest impulse towards the scientific and rational clarity of human thought; and it is again this rationality which determines the disillusioned and responsible eye of bourgeois ethics, its pragmatism and the spirit of capitalism. All bourgeois revolutions sooner or later formed an alliance with the reforming spirit of Protestant ethics, in the context of the respective monotheistic traditions, until the secular evolution which has now become global.

In medicine, some degree of a renewed sense of *kaloskagathos* is constantly though unconsciously requested, especially by certain patients and doctors, who know that the beautiful can contribute decisively to the development of an enriched perception of illness and treatment. Doctors and paramedics need beauty, not least because it can help them to avoid betraying themselves and the trust placed in them by their patients – not to submit their souls to the mechanical routine of the world of action. Hospitals need beauty, which would already be therapeutic in itself; but above all, patients need it and seek it in minute details, in relations, in the changing nature of the expressions of the faces and words of those they love.

And here I would hazard a suggestion: why don't the great architects build hospitals to be not simply hospitals but temples of beauty and of dignity in suffering? It would be possible, with the help of doctors and patients, to found a new branch of architecture as a science and discipline of hospitality for the suffering and their treatment. The quest for the form of such a hospital could become in itself the central core of reflection on the meaning of illness, in the places where death most frequently occurs.

Perseus's courage: the indirect vision

Postmodern human beings tend to free themselves critically of identification with their own conscience as a metaphor of the world, but this may prevent them from continuing to explore themselves and to appreciate, free of reverential fear, their own experience of meaning and their heritage of myths, meanings and narratives. If the human being's innate creative stimulus is not cultivated, it can generate monsters – titans that collapse under the weight of the world's opaqueness, which they have not clarified.

Nietzsche, in *Thus Spake Zarathustra*, alludes to the perils of this weight: 'For unto him who possesseth it, all that is possessed is well hidden; and of all treasure pits, one's own is digged out last. Thus the spirit of gravity causeth it to be.' And he adds:

> Man is difficult to discover, and hardest of all unto himself. Often the spirit lieth over the soul. Thus the spirit of gravity causeth it to be.

But he hath discovered himself who saith: 'This is *my* good and evil.'
Thereby he hath made mute the mole and dwarf who saith: 'Good for
all, evil for all'.[11]

If the human spirit becomes light, it must remain firmly anchored to the
reality of its own life and time, but not one-sidedly identified with it. Such
an active awareness knows how to avoid identifying with the communal
rhetoric; it learns to scent the risk of its ideas being infected by the collective
dimension of mass society; for the archaic forces of the group, the impulse
towards the inflation and dissociation of personality in the name of collective identification, always remain latent in it. It is the perception of form,
lightness and respect for the flow of time, rather than content itself, that
first sense this and highlight the danger of a collective tendency. As common
sense suggests, excitement, insistence and haste are premonitory signs of it.
When the ego does not fear its own knowledge, it becomes a slave to it, and
its own attitude reduces value, turns discourse into idle chatter.

Jung, in the Red Book, may have revealed the reason why the 'divine
madness' of the years of his visionary introversion, his 'creative illness', did
not lead to psychopathology. He describes subjective identification with
the spirit of the abyss as a sick delusion, but applies the same description
to the practice of limiting oneself to the surface, exchanging absolute individual freedom of judgement for the dominant attitude of the *Zeitgeist*,
the spirit of the times. If individuals want to avoid the spectre of madness, they
are compelled to speak both to the spirit of their time and to the spirit of the
depths; in order to speak to the one, while remaining themselves, they have
to continue their dialogue with the other.[12]

Here lightness is presented, as it is by Calvino in the first of his *Memos
for the Next Millennium*, as a value and a task; for the spirit can become
as light as Perseus on Mercury's winged *talaria*. Like Calvino, we all have
moments when the world seems to turn to stone, as in a process of petrifica-
tion in varying degrees that spares no aspect of life, as if it were not possible
to avoid the Medusa's inexorable gaze. Only a hero like Perseus, flying on
winged sandals given him by Mercury, supported by the winds and clouds,
can manage, with his lightness, to look at Medusa's reflected image in the
bronze shield. Only with an indirect gaze can he face and defeat the world's
opacity and heaviness by decapitating the monster (see Figure 6.2).

In our society, Medusa might represent the weight of the literalism and
unilateral extroversion of our times. But as Calvino writes, the question of
the relationship between Perseus and Medusa does not end with the Gorgon's decapitation; out of her body springs a winged horse, Pegasus, which,

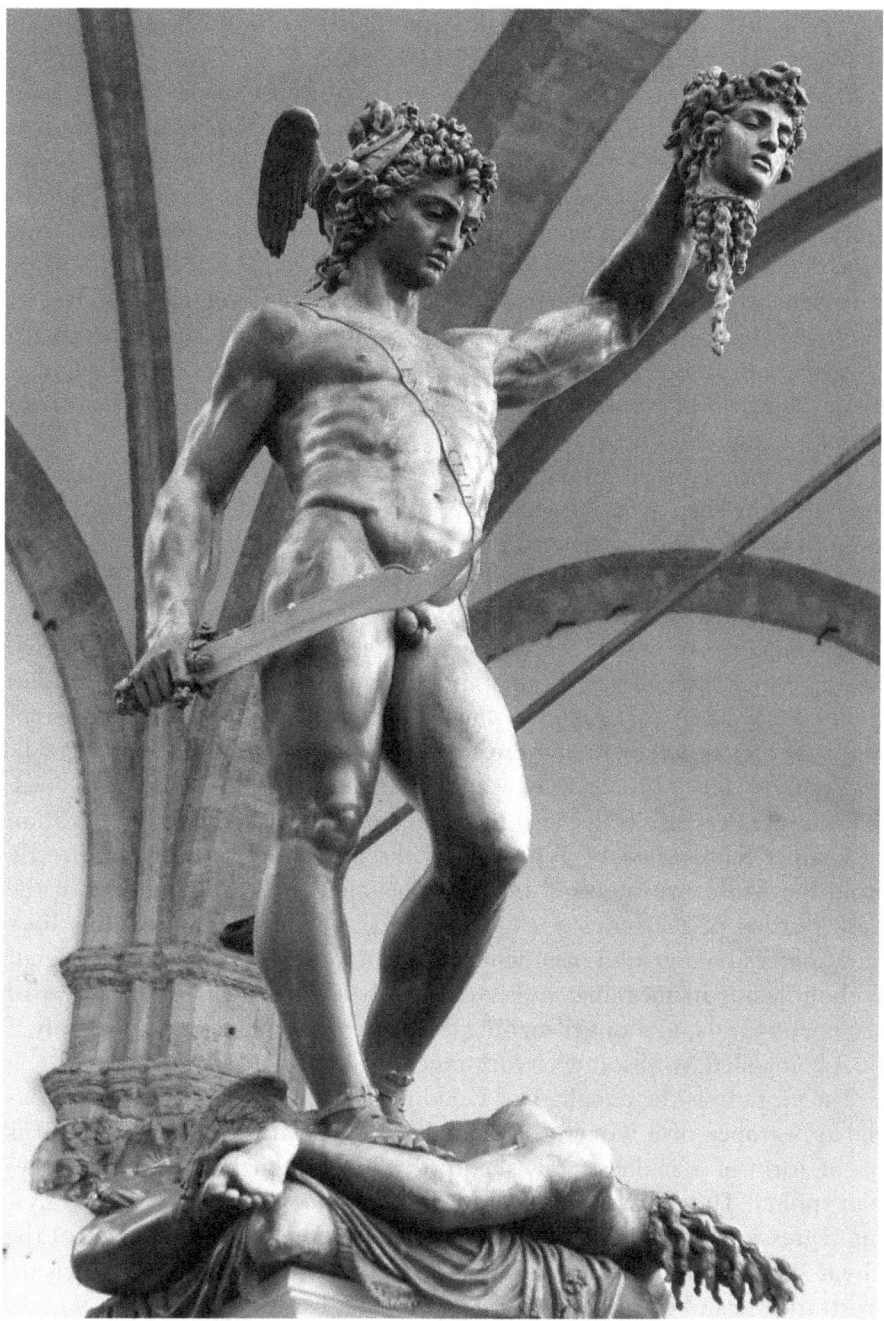

Figure 6.2 Perseus with the Head of Medusa. Benvenuto Cellini. Loggia dei Lanzi, Florence.
© Marie-Lan Nguyen – Wikimedia Commons.

with one blow of its hoof, will make water gush out of the rock on Mount Helicon – the spring from which the Muses drink.[13]

Perseus will always carry Medusa's head with him, in the magic pouch given him by the Naiads of Seriphos (the *kibisis*). This gesture entails a great, irreversible effort – today mainly an individual and subjective one – that of always carrying on your shoulders the weight of reality, which, in every sense, follows you, clings behind you, like an object slung over your shoulder, on your back.

Perseus succeeds in mastering that terrible face by keeping it hidden, as previously he had defeated it by looking at it in the mirror. Perseus's strength always lies in a rejection of the direct gaze, but not in a rejection of the reality of the world of monsters in which it is his lot to live – a reality he carries with him, and takes upon himself as his own burden.[14]

This onerous but necessary task represents both the weight of the awareness that has been acquired – a weapon to be used against the enemy only as a last resort – and a warning against the constant danger of relapsing into the temptations of the literal world view, of fundamentalisms and ideologies.

At an individual level Medusa represents the unconscious, a regression to dependence; in killing the monster, the hero overcomes his fear of the feminine, of the fearsome mother, and abandons childhood; the hero dies to himself (*in a sense, he is himself Medusa, an innate misogynous internal image of the feminine*), and after the decapitation he becomes mature, willing to carry with him the weight and creative richness of the unconscious. The mature Perseus's tragic vision is linked on the one hand to the elevation of instinct represented by Pegasus and the possibility of drawing directly from the Muses' spring; and on the other hand to his taking care of the dark burden of the monster's head of hair, a chimera that contains life's dark material secret, and from which it will never be possible to free oneself without losing its meaning. So Perseus will be able to lay bare the power of the unconscious, in a direct manner, but only in extreme situations, only if he is compelled by absolute circumstances of life.

The Gorgon is the daughter of Echidna, a chimera whose upper half has the appearance of a woman of matchless beauty and whose lower half is in the form of a snake. It was she, too, who gave birth to Oedipus's Theban sphinx. These archaic figures represent the constant risk of a paralysing regression to maternal dependence, the fearsome, devouring face of the Great Mother – the mother to whom no shadows, imperfections, criticisms, frustrations can be attributed; or the pseudo-altruistic mother who will do anything for her child, but in fact tries to preserve a positive image of herself; or the mother who does not allow her child to go away, but forces him or her to realize the greatness that is the condition of her love. Or, simply, regression to the omnipotence of infinite, fusional desire, which is never satisfied, but condemned to the unhappiness of those who are incapable of achieving 'balance' in the exercise of their virtue; Perseus as the hero of self-knowledge, capable of an inward gaze.

What is the link between the myth of Perseus and medicine? Perseus is an example of the courage of a light, indirect vision, even in the face of the terrible monsters of the human being's inner world. He is a hero who makes introversion an instrument of knowledge and a precious creative force, which he can use in the outer world, an instrument endowed with far greater resources than the concretist approach. Perseus's perspective is one that should encourage the public of patients to reconsider the uncritically idealized image of the technological hero and not to underestimate the real practical and emotional knowledge of the doctor they have in front of them.

The new sense of reality acquired by Perseus after the killing of Medusa is an active effort of awareness. From the intermediate zone between the inner and outer worlds, between the ego and the unconscious, it realizes in actions the forms of the reality of the psyche. Only the encounter with reality and the curbing of the tension of this encounter can be creative. The point of departure is a place of the imagination, an intermediate space, which is differentiated from the 'world of fantasy' precisely by the absence of any dissociative component to take the place of reality, and by its light bearing, prone to playfulness and laughter, in the conscious world. The opacity and static heaviness of the world, and the spectre of permanence, of fixity, are transformed, acquiring a dynamic, musical value, which is channelled into the effort of consciousness. It is a movement that starts from the archaic and typical richness of the self, humanity's common heritage, and determines an enrichment and reinforcement of the dominion of consciousness. The ego acquires significance from its virtue or *daimon* only if it becomes strong enough to set its own limit (rather than having it imposed from outside), which is translated into its own moral law (immune to fundamentalisms). By knowing itself, it can set a limit to its own virtue, realizing itself in the propensity to happiness (*eu-daimonia*) that is discussed by Salvatore Natoli.[15]

In psychoanalytic jargon this can mean integrating into the conscious structure a healthy superego capable of offering the subject the gift of living; structuring progressively, through experience, not only the distinction between the dimensions of the self and the object, but also the contrasting emotional valences of the self and the object.

The ambivalence of the inner and outer objectival needs becomes acceptable when the complexity and richness of the world are interiorized and articulated in an individual narrative which also embraces the dissonances, the 'irreconcilables', without demanding an impossible reconciliation. This process causes the unknown to lose its sense of menace for the consciousness, and the ego to acquire a degree of ironic detachment, the smile. There is in this a wholly human compensation for the instinct of attack/flight/freeze, for the paranoid tendency innate in the human being (the persecutory nature of the obscure, unconscious sides of a distorted superego or of a primitive, overwhelming threat of annihilation), tending towards an extreme simplification of reality, towards the fixed idea which generates the objective absolute hero. This can be replaced by a detached vision, whose moral perspective is enriched by having seen the dark spaces of the mind, the madness inherent in human existence and the necessary deflation of omnipotence.

In human suffering there can be a superstructural element, interpretative and imaginative at the same time, capable of amplifying indefinitely the psychic perception of pain. Of the three Cerberus-heads of suffering, one is that of exposure to the other, as a result of which the subject, being ill and in pain, feels threatened by his or her condition of disability and dependence; it exposes the individual to an undesired and significant sense of vulnerability. Then there is a second head, that of deficiency, of the impossibility of a response commensurate with need, of indifference, negligence, pretence, disgust or denial. The first head is related to the experience of vulnerability, the second to the experience of powerlessness, both of which alter the self's integrity. Each of these produces a sense of degradation, shame and loss of dignity. But the most ferocious is the third, that of a compulsive collusion with one's own suffering, which is related to trauma. In the innermost being it turns against itself an element of sadism that is innate in every human being – and perhaps in some other primates too – which is a product of the entirely human tension between unnatural ferocity and an inexhaustible capacity for suffering – between imperialism and passivity.

Such psychic pain, when repeated, generates structured depression and anxiety, thus modifying the brain, through the compulsive repetition of a foreclosed narrative of suffering and violence and the internalization of this predatory 'surplus'. Such a destructive drive, when not 'acted out' in the external world (an important source of violence), can run along the route of the somato-psychic matrix, thus contributing to the creation and maintenance of many diseases, attacking the host's psyche or soma, as has been documented by several authors, such as Van der Kolk in his study of trauma, *The Body Keeps the Score*, or Joyce McDougall in her *Theatres of the Body*, and Donald Kalsched, in his *The Inner World of Trauma: Archetypal Defences of the Personal Spirit*.[16]

Unfortunately, the third Cerberus-head can sometimes collude with a potentially sadistic degeneration of the doctor's medicalizing unconscious – the darkest shadow of Asclepius. In the transition between wounding and dying that is essential to the medical act, pragmatism can become detrimental to intelligence and compassion in managing the great prevalence of unrecognized traumatic disorders. Under the pressure of collective shame and denial with regard to the issue of trauma and its ubiquity, the enormous market-driven diffusion of psychiatric drugs, or in former times the systematic use of electric shock therapy or frontal lobotomy, become examples of how this sadistic shadow of the doctor has been acted out. This also provides an important explanation of the stubborn attachment to concretistic defences shown by many patients affected by somatic ailments. Perseus's courage, and in particular his approach after he has confronted the terrifying Medusa-face of madness, help us to understand, manage and perhaps cure each of these three perversions of human suffering.

From another perspective, Perseus's courage in the face of pain can also be seen in the patients' reticence, in the capacity for self-restraint, which preserves the individual form of the person's being by dissimulating suffering and, as far as possible, feigning joy. In the face of the dissolution represented by illness, the patient suffers inwardly, but keeps within the limit and eschews any mournful tone, does not become fixated on a depressive nostalgia for the lost object. As Natoli recalls in *L'Esperienza del Dolore* (The Experience of Pain),[17] the time of exercising the great simulation of art becomes a discipline of life; real joy blends with the simulated variety, irony attenuates melancholy, a cheerful attitude lightens the uncertainty of the days. A melancholy sense of exclusion from life, an oblique and absent gaze, a fixation of unlived life, give way to the fulfilment of the still intact and latent potential of a person's being. This implies transcending the pure technical indication, a deliberate transition to the intermediate zone of the limit of all scientific knowledge and therefore within what has determined one's diagnostic and therapeutic experience. It is a going beyond, towards an openness to a wider, indefinable sphere which has presupposed the limit and transcends it. Perseus, who does not look at life's heaviness directly, but carries it with him, loads it on to his back and bears its weight inwardly, is a good symbol of the tension of reticence in illness. Even the functionalism of appearances becomes acceptable in the context of such an awareness. In striving to understand the lifestyle congenial to one who has found their own measure, the discipline gradually delineates it. People have become able to bear suffering by inventing and experiencing the intense joy of moments, even of their last remaining ones, whatever the pain. Modern medicine can offer great help to anyone capable of such courage, and this fact has certainly contributed to its diffusion and confirmation in history.

Notes

1 Camus 1942, p. 9.
2 Rilke 1929, p. 33.
3 Ibidem, p. 34.
4 Zoja 2000, pp. 89–90.
5 Ibidem, p. 83.
6 Ibidem.
7 See Hillman 1981, pp. 11–17 on the unitary seat of imagination, and pp. 18–25, on Harvey.
8 In Italian *Il fuoco di Sant'Antonio* is the normal colloquial term for *herpes zoster*, or shingles. In English, for historical reasons, the name 'St Anthony's Fire' came to be used for two different skin infections, erysipelas and ergotism.
9 Augustine, Book X, chapter 6, pp. 582–583:

> What now do I love, whenas I love thee? Not the beauty of any corporal thing, not the order of times, not the brightness of the light, which to behold is so gladsome to our eyes; not the pleasant melodies of songs of all kinds, not the fragrant smell of flowers, and ointment, and spices; not manna and honey, nor any fair limbs that are so acceptable to fleshly embracements. I love none of these things, whenas I love my God: and yet I love a certain kind of light, and a kind of voice, and a kind of fragrancy, and a kind of meat, and a kind of embracement, whenas I love my God; who is both the light, and the voice, and the sweet smell, and the meat, and the embracement of my inner man; where that light shineth unto my soul which no place can receive, that voice soundeth which time deprives me not of, and that fragrancy smelleth which no wind scatters, and that meat tasteth, which eating devours not, and that embracement clingeth to me which satiety divorceth not. This is it which I love, whenas I love my God.

10 Zoja 2007a, p. 9:

> For the modern mentality, with its abstract and defining categories, the contraposition between ethics and aesthetics is clear. Aesthetics can remain personal and relative; ethics inherently strives toward the absolute. Therefore we can do without aesthetics, but cannot escape ethics. The Greeks, to whom we owe the *definitions* of both ethics and aesthetics, would have rejected their *separation*. There were no written codes that defined beauty or goodness. But there was a general consensus about both, and also a consensus about the fact that they belong together. The two were different expressions of the same quality – excellence – to such an extent that their kinship came to be expressed by combining two words in one: by a single word, *kalokagathia* = beauty-and-goodness. Both corresponded to the longing for something divine. Yes, one could describe them, in the manner of an abstract exercise, as two distinct things. But in concrete reality it was assumed that they always came together – as two faces of the same coin – because the longing that animates them, the soul's research for elevation, is inherently one. In the sense proposed by Martin Buber, these two ideas were *Grundworte* (basic words): concepts that perform their function only if related as a dyad, never alone.

'As Thomas Mann had noted, Nietzsche was, in a brilliant synthesis, the first psychologist and the most tenacious antimodernist, for saying simply this: the aesthetic heritage – the true heritage of the Greeks – has been forgotten, but

cannot be eliminated' (Zoja 2007b, p. 20 of the Italian text – English version by the translator of this volume).
11 Nietzsche 1883–85, pp. 280–281.
12 Jung 1915–30, p. 150:

> This is how I overcame madness. If you do not know what divine madness is, suspend judgment and wait for the fruits. But know that there is a divine madness which is nothing other than the overpowering of the spirit of this time through the spirit of the depths. Speak then of sick delusion when the spirit of the depths can no longer stay down and forces a man to speak in tongues instead of in human speech, and makes him believe that he himself is the spirit of the depths. But also speak of sick delusion when the spirit of this time does not leave a man and forces him to see only the surface, to deny the spirit of the depths and to take himself for the spirit of the times. The spirit of this time is ungodly; the spirit of the depths is ungodly; balance is godly.

13 Calvino 1988, p. 5.
14 Calvino 1988, p. 3.
15 Natoli 2003.
16 Van der Kolk 2014; McDougall 1989; and Kalsched 1996.
17 Natoli 1986, pp. 155–157.

Bibliography

Augustine, *Confessions*, translated by William Watts, London: John Norton for John Partridge, 1631.

Calvino, Italo (1988), *Lezioni Americane. Sei Proposte per il Prossimo Millennio. Six Memos for the Next Millennium: The Charles Eliot Norton Lectures, 1985–1986*, translated by Patrick Creagh, London: Penguin Modern Classics, 1993.

Camus, Albert (1942), *Le Mythe de Sisyphe*, Paris: Gallimard, 1942.

Hillman, James (1981), *The Thought of the Heart and the Soul of the World*, Woodstock, CT: Spring Publications, 1997.

Jung, Carl Gustav (1915–30), *The Red Book: Liber Novus: A Reader's Edition*, edited by Sonu Shamdasani, preface by Ulrich Hoerni, translated by Mark Kyburz, John Peck, and Sonu Shamdasani, New York & London: W.W. Norton & Co., 2009.

Kalsched, Donald (1996), *The Inner World of Trauma: Archetypal Defences of the Personal Spirit*, London: Routledge, 1996.

McDougall, Joyce (1989), *Theatres of the Body: A Psychoanalytic Approach to Psychosomatic Illness*, New York: W.W. Norton & Co., 1989.

Natoli, Salvatore (1986), *L'Esperienza del Dolore: Le Forme del Patire nella Cultura Occidentale. The Experience of Pain: The Forms of Suffering in Western Culture*, Milan: Feltrinelli, 2008.

Natoli, Salvatore (2003), *La Felicità: Saggio di Teoria degli Affetti. Happiness: An Essay on the Theory of Affects*, Milan: Feltrinelli, 2003.

Nietzsche, Friedrich (1883–85), *Also Sprach Zarathustra: Ein Buch für Alle und Kleinen. Thus Spake Zarathustra: A Book for All and None*, translated by Alexander Tille, London: The Macmillan Co., 1896.

Rilke, Rainer Maria (1929), *Briefe an Einen Jungen Dichter*, Leipzig: Insel-Verlag, 1932.

Van der Kolk, Bessel A. (2014), *The Body Keeps the Score: Brain, Mind, and Body in the Healing of Trauma*, New York: Penguin Books, 2014.

Zoja, Luigi (2000), *Il Gesto di Ettore: Preistoria, Storia, Attualità e Scomparsa del Padre. The Father: Historical, Psychological and Cultural Perspectives*, translated by Henry Martin, East Sussex & Philadelphia: Brunner Routledge, 2001.

Zoja, Luigi (2007a), *Ethics and Analysis: Philosophical Perspectives and Their Application in Therapy*, College Station, TX: Texas A&M University Press, 2007.

Zoja, Luigi (2007b), *Giustizia e Bellezza*, Turin: Bollati Boringhieri, 2007.

Part III

Life hanging by a thread

Chapter 7

Illness as an experience of the soul

The experience of illness and *furor sanandi*

Once the 'acute phase' of a serious illness has passed, the violent reactions of the psyche to the narrow escape from death generates intense conditionings and constellates often unconscious meanings, in the form of images or fantasies, which are channelled by the collective consciousness, so that this becomes an effective container for them. During this phase, rationalization is a fairly common defence mechanism; sometimes denial or splitting occurs. In this process the doctor may make a prudent contribution, sensitive to the processing of defensive reactions by the patient. It is more common for the doctor to choose a neutral position, fomenting the technological automatism of treatment, by encouraging patients to use their own faculties of processing with little or no help, and strengthening their defences, when these facilitate the execution of the treatment programme. The over-medicalization of society is in my opinion increased by the prevalence of this approach. A concretistic obsession with pills, or sometimes a one-sided rejection of them, an insistence on continuing treatment or rejecting it passively, added to the oppressive sense of the burden one is laying on society, are all driven by a failure to process the experience of illness and the treatment that is applied.

It is not surprising, however, that the considerable improvement in health and quality of life provided by technological medical progress is not perceived as such by many patients. Although modern medicine is incomparably more effective than in any other period, the doctor is not accorded the same unconditional trust that used to be placed in the family doctor. My profession, as a hospital cardiologist in one of the public hospitals of Milan, gives me daily experience of the remarkable effectiveness of technological medical operations for the survival of heart attack patients. Rapid recovery tends to lead to denial or repression of the experience of illness. Therapeutic success in acute cases has also caused a gradual increase in the evolution towards chronic illness, owing to the fact that an increasing number of patients survives until the advanced stages of heart disease. These patients suffering from chronic heart failure are faced with frequent hospitalizations and limitations on their bodily functions (and quality of life), the growing socio-economic cost of which places an increasing burden on the health service, and leads to greater social exclusion, as well as loneliness, anxiety and depression (at least a fifth of heart patients are affected by a major anxious or depressive disorder). In such patients, who are more in contact with their own vulnerability and dependence, I often sense a deeper, sometimes unexpressed thirst, which expresses itself, despite all their attempts to deny it, in a gentle humour, free from absolute expectations. It is an approach which perhaps once found an echo and sublimation in the great container of tradition, through religion, myths and folk tales.

The Italian journalist Enzo Biagi once asked the author and film director Pier Paolo Pasolini: 'You said that we become more cheerful as we grow older; why is that?' Pasolini replied: 'Because we have a shorter future, and therefore fewer hopes, and that is a great joy'.[1] As has already been mentioned, having less 'hope', according to Hillman – in the sense of abandoning pride, its omnipotent aspect – cures people of their dogged determination to live. Hope, the only evil still trapped in Pandora's vase, is the most forgivable of evils, being interwoven with the instinct of survival, but it does nothing active to improve the quality of life. Hope in our times seems fixated on an infinite longing, an insatiable bulimia of desire. Is this blindness the punishment that the gods inflicted on the human race, concealed under the magnificent forms of Pandora – that of drifting aimlessly between the passive acceptance of one's misfortune and a desire for a modicum of power, between endurance and the constant temptation to enjoy the enticement of easy satisfaction?

Nowadays, after the 'death of God' announced by Nietzsche,[2] inner transcendence is often achieved by the rational shortcut of eliminating the symptom on the physical level. In an extreme vision, the doctor appears as the agent of an impersonal institution, entrusted with the task of restoring the patient 'to working order' as an individual, a cog in the social machinery provided by public healthcare. Patients are led to project their intimate needs for transcendence on to the screen of reason, which shows them a functional image, but also offers them collective containment, by promising to alleviate both their suffering and their solitude at the same time. Although this promise is often fulfilled, it also eliminates the need for a reflective process, targeting the discovery of a deeper level of meaning. The hospital system presses for illness not to be felt as an experience of the limited nature of the human condition, but as a temporary obstacle to be overcome under the social pressure of role identity and the economy, so as to be able to return to the linear time of productivity. Thus medicine asserts, under the cloak of its own real empirical efficacy, the tyranny of chronological time in the life of the individual, even in such timeless moments.

In these public places, the hospitals, as in other environments, the dimension of subjectivity, and therefore of relationships, which is so important in medicine, is easily eliminated by the requirements of functionalism. The often unconscious *furor agendi* of functional efficiency replaces and eliminates any possibility of authentic reflection, and becomes a *furor sanandi* of the conscious attitude. The doctor's relationship with the patient is simplified and impoverished by the reification of the body, in the name of a higher nobility of the purpose, while the uncomfortable effort to enter into a relationship, within the egalitarian context of an intersubjective dyad, is reduced to the minimum. This simplification, when it does not imply a heroic vision of medicine, satisfies the need to remain firmly anchored to one's own role identity, removing fear and the inability of many doctors to examine their own dark inner spaces. However, it is precisely in supportive relationships that are delineated in such a one-sided manner that the little-explored dark spaces become so many opportunities for a constellation of the doctor's shadow.

In clinical practice I have often wondered how it is possible to welcome the gifts of technology, while accepting the implicit deflation of the experience of meaning that the technological operation entails, and at the same time to safeguard the cognitive potential of the experience of illness, of the imminence of mortality as a vital process of the psyche, which consciously stimulates and enriches one's own vision of the world. On other occasions, I have found myself feeling sceptical in the face of the ease with which patients also submit to the pursuance of medical treatment as an impersonal routine, reluctant as they often are to confront their own emotions and the conscious experience of their own vulnerability. I wondered whether that research and that reflective ability might not represent a 'treatment' for the soul, and whether the doctor might not encourage this critical and participatory function, so that it could be naturally integrated into the process of 'treatment', in a manner that was independent, yet intimately connected with the experiences of the body.[3] The answer is probably that both these positions, that of doubt and that of trust, are legitimate. On the one hand, the denial of death is inherent in that container of the collective consciousness which has, through science, elevated the power of humankind, including the lower levels of society in prosperity (that unprecedented historical event which, albeit with tragic limitations in the so-called third world, is spreading from the West to the rest of humanity). On the other hand, the lack of interest in the question of significance might simply be due to a widespread indifference in contemporary society to the great questions traditionally posed by philosophy, which have now become the domain of science, as mankind is inebriated by the expectation of gaining access to a prosperity that has no precedent in history. But the subject of death is present in the souls of all individuals and their families more or less consciously, just like that of sense and nonsense, from the moment of birth. Doctors should draw on the long philosophical tradition of their art, resisting the automatism of normative mechanisms, and not miss the great cognitive and educational opportunity that is offered to them every day, not only with regard to the sick and society, but also with regard to themselves.

Technology, in its alliance with power, actively promotes the doctors' 'fall' into the darkness of their own shadows, into the moral indifference of their own 'technological' unconscious, which, if it is not revealed, becomes contrary to any individuation. The darkest shadow of the medical profession is the fact that it has shirked the task of making the moral and human implications of technological predominance conscious and restoring them to free will.

In the world of functionalism and unlimited consumption, death concretized in the present and transformed into a collective taboo, and at the same time repressed by the omnipotence of the technological gesture of treatment, will re-emerge as guilt, just like any inability, inadequacy and vulnerability.

Luigi Zoja puts it as follows:

> If God has been removed from the heavens and re-incarnated into human aspirations that are no less infinite, death too, removed from sight, has likewise been displaced and not eliminated. It makes its re-appearance in the interior of the individual, assuming the guise of states of depression that escape all rational explanation. At the core of such an absence of *élan vital* lies a sense of absolute guilt which again, in rational terms, seems wholly unmotivated; it accompanies the perception of living a life that knows of no sufficient justification for continuing to exist. Guilt, as an interior feeling of which the causes remain imprecise, is a survival of the death we deny and the soul we devalue; so it makes unconscious allusion to the traditional figure of the death of the soul. The feeling of bearing a guilt of which the origins remain inexplicable finds no referent in specific responsibilities; it refers to the ancestral terror of spiritual demise.[4]

Not only depression, but also the numerous psychosomatic manifestations of our age, probably express the return of the repressed sense of limit, exercising through the soma what the aspiration to the unlimited no longer encounters in the psyche, which often turns one-sidedly towards the outer world. In this sense, physical illness may have a distinct compensatory effect, recalling, through the body, the limit that is announced in the body's illness as destiny. It is no coincidence that about one-fifth of the entire population of cardiopathic patients are afflicted by a clinically significant depressive disorder. Depression and heart disease represent, together, the main cause of disability in developed societies and it is predicted that this will be true on a global scale by 2030.[5]

In the Ancient Egyptian *Book of the Dead* (Figure 7.1), the traditional figure of the death of the soul takes the form of the chimerical monster Ammit, part lion, part hippopotamus, part crocodile. Every soul (Ba, in the form of a bird) was accompanied into the Duat (the underworld, according to the Egyptians' religion) by Anubis, the guardian of the dead and companion of souls. Their hearts were weighed in the 'room of two truths' on a balance guarded by Anubis. Under the wise supervision of Thot, the god of writing, the dead person's heart was placed on one side of the balance and Maat's feather on the other. Maat, the goddess of cosmic order, corresponded to grace, truth and justice, which comprised the very architecture of the cosmos (*kosmos*, or 'ornament', which would later become the 'universe' of monotheism). Maat was represented as a winged woman, with an ostrich feather in her hair. If a person's heart did not prove to be as light as Maat's feather, it was devoured by Ammit and could not make the journey to the Duat. The condemnation of the soul was connected with sin and guilt, as is confirmed

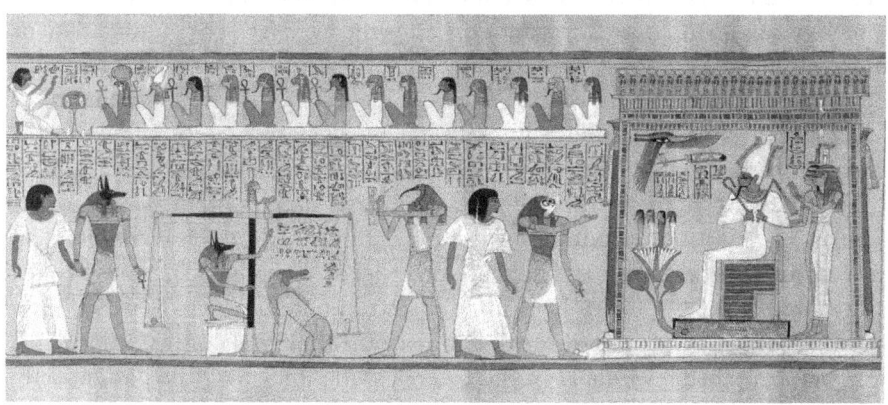

Figure 7.1 Book of the Dead of Hunefer, Sheet 3, Egypt, 19th Dynasty, c. 1275 B.C.E., 44.5 x 30.7 cm, Thebes, Egypt.

by the hymns of the text which list the reprehensible actions that can make the heart 'heavier'. This link between death and guilt also recalls the child, when it traces the primal terror of not-being to a sense of guilt. Only the heart's lightness enables the soul to identify itself, by recognizing, at a transpersonal level, its own position in the world. There is a dual movement here: only if human beings become containers and limits of their own virtue does that virtue make them share in something which recognizes and elevates them at the same time; in the absence of this simultaneously ethical and aesthetic movement, the unique and precious trace of that individuality does not remain; instead, it perishes for ever, dissolving in the undifferentiated. A similar concept is expressed by the idea that we do not possess our virtues or our *daimon*, but rather the contrary: it is they that possess us.

Solitude in serious illness

In serious illness, when there is an imminent danger of death, the body rebels with all its strength, activating the physiological systems responsible for maintaining homeostasis. This translates into a violent alarm system of the organism, manifested in a crescendo of psychic suffering, panic in the face of the appalling prospect of death. The unparalleled violence of a direct threat to existence is inevitably deeply traumatic. In the most serious cases, medicine deals with this problem by inducing the patient's unconsciousness by pharmacological means. Nevertheless, in this case the memory of the progressive decline until the collapse that preceded anaesthesia and intubation remains. Only a minority (about one-fifth) of survivors have no memory at all of the time they spent in intensive care. Moreover, a few months after their recovery, about one patient in five is affected by post-traumatic stress disorder, whose appearance seems to be correlated to the length of the periods of wakefulness during intubation.[6]

Patients, rendered completely voiceless by the presence of the endotracheal tube, are unable to express meaning in words, but cough, oppose things that are done to them, feel pain, thirst, hunger, itching, and often squirm . . . their state of consciousness is fluctuating, the oneiric activity preserved, and they cannot communicate their needs verbally, their voice evokes suffocated silence. This leads in some cases to an intense introversion, even during moments of consciousness, and periods of mental confusion or delirium are described, especially in the elderly, sometimes with the patient only seemingly calm, the classic 'patient who doesn't make a fuss', but behind whose frozen facial expression images of great agitation are likely to be hidden. The often fragmentary remembrance of these moments seems to determine the subsequent onset of post-traumatic stress. There are usually brief periods of spontaneous awakening, or anaesthetists may 'switch' patients' minds on and off pharmacologically when they attempt to 'wean them off' the ventilator or various other mechanical devices.

On waking up, patients discover indelible signs on their bodies of the experience they have been through, signs which faithfully preserve the memory of the great 'subversion' they have suffered. Both conscious and unconscious factors underlie the effect of the experience of illness's 'attack' on psychic life with the return to consciousness. At a subjective level, they correspond to a sense of the ineffable and intangible nature of the alienating experience the patient has just had.

The psyche's normal reaction to an intolerable experience is to withdraw from the scene of the damage; when this is not possible through the induction of the state of unconsciousness, the individual is unable to ward off the experience with the normal psychic defences, and is forced to seek dissociation from it. There may be a separation between the various tonalities of the experience of the world, such as the cognitive aspect, the affective aspect, corporeal sensitivity and the imagination, which can no longer be experienced in a harmonious and unitary manner. According to Kalsched, the author of the only real study of trauma from the archetypal point of view, a fragmentation of the integrity of psychic life is associated with the emergence of inner defences, which are archaic and archetypal, because they are not personally developed and controllable.[7] These defences, replacing the outer damage even when this has ended, remove the 'unthinkable' emotion associated with the traumatic experience. This happens in such a way as to cause a complete separation between the conscious experience and the essential nucleus of the individual's integrity, between life as a cluster of conscious experiences and that essential thread of inner sensations, images and representations in which the whole individual is expressed, in which the centre of gravity that Jung calls the self is manifested. The dissociation prevents any harmony in this process; it alters the process profoundly, generating a dominant traumatogenic imago which will tend to perpetuate the experience of the trauma. Although its initial purpose is the absolute protection of the fundamental nucleus of the self, which is indispensable for survival, it eventually turns against the individual, as in autoimmune diseases, when the defence mechanism evades control and attacks the host.

Similarly, if patients who survive a very serious bout of illness – so serious as to require invasive assistance – do not activate adequate defensive reactions which might enable them to work through and integrate the experience, they will react with extreme anxiety to the slightest symptom that re-evokes it. For example, if a person who has suffered a heart attack in the past feels a non-specific chest pain, their fear of the self's disintegration is concretized in that pain, and focused on the heart. This reaction also occurs in people who have not previously had any heart problems, proof that psychic contagion is facilitated both by the emotional impact of the heart as a symbol and by the widespread occurrence of heart disease in the population. The risk, especially in acute traumatic illness, is that the patient will not succeed in containing the archaic defences that amplify suffering, making the experience of the disease completely irreconcilable with the nucleus of the personality. It is in this context that medical technology most clearly performs its salvific and numinous role.[8] Typically embodied in the surgeon, it not only 'saves' patients from death, it enables them to 'postpone' the very prospect of their mortality, by giving them a world in which the victory of good over evil is the only vehicle of experience, without any possible ambiguities or qualifications. This brings us back to the heroic conception of present-day medicine.

The symbolic function is that vital faculty of the psyche which tends not to eliminate contrast but to overcome it, by realizing a higher unity in the symbol. It has a profound resonance from the individual's experience with the soul, which arises out of the imagination of the other and constantly influences the tone and colour of a person's perception of the world. Awareness (in this sense neither solely rational nor solely emotional) restores the person to his or her fundamental reality (not reduced to the mechanical nature or the purely egoic environment of the exchange), bringing into play the cognitive function that emotions and intuition contain. The mere sight of a branch or a flower through the light of a window can stimulate this vital function and provide a point of departure. This function of imaginative dialogue with the outer world is universally present and active in all human beings. Through it, the individual realizes a continual synthesis of two opposing polarities: on the one hand the intra-psychic elements – such as rationality and emotionality, thought and eros, consciousness and unconsciousness – and on the other the two terms of the relationship, the 'I' and the 'you': in our case, the patient on one side and the therapist, the doctor or (more often) the nurse on the other. In this regard, as Jung said:

> The unrelated human being lacks wholeness, for he cannot achieve wholeness only through the soul, and the soul cannot exist without its other side, which is always found in a 'You'. Wholeness is a combination of I and You and these show themselves to be parts of a transcendent unity whose nature can only be grasped symbolically.[9]

Architects who design intensive therapy rooms could perhaps bear such considerations in mind, providing the eye with an opening towards the outside, access to relatives, a view of the sky, trees or meadows, and the possibility of observing the changes of day and night not only on a clock face.

The doctor or nurse should try to guide the patient's lost, sometimes almost blank gaze, with its abyss of questioning and non-sense, accepting the inner conflict and the sense of powerlessness, the sadness, the despair, the aggression, trying to offer containment or listen to the expression of overflowing emotions. They will be able to do all this if they keep the channels of intuition open, in a dialogue, even if it is only a silent one, in which they treat the patient not as something other than themselves, but as a fellow human being, opening themselves to the emotions in a manner free from prejudice, not allowing a reductive attitude to get in the way of the relationship. The premise is immediate trust or distrust, at first sight, at the first meeting. In this regard, Eugenio Borgna affirms, with reference to the psychiatric patient, that

> emotions flood over us, anguish drags us into the maelstrom of experiences that border on nonsense and nothingness, sadness strikes us dumb and isolates us, aggression overwhelms us, and yet the possibility of entering into a relationship with another person, where there is trust, performs a radical therapeutic signification – stemming, even at a first meeting, the overflowing emotions: diseased emotions.[10]

Like the mental patient, a person suffering from a serious, acute or chronic physical condition is sorely tried by emotions. It is therefore important to understand the therapeutic value of the involvement of the doctor or nurse's subjectivity, particularly perhaps in the context of *serious* organic disease, and especially for the more vulnerable patient. If they use empathy and open dialogue, even of a non-verbal kind, the therapists will prevent the patient from being swallowed up in solitude, maintaining his or her contact with outer reality. For this to happen, they must themselves be psychologically able to integrate ambivalences, by preserving contact both with the patient and with their own emotions, and being prepared both to welcome and to contain their own feelings, as well as those of the patient, without debasing the soul of either party in the cold mirror of indifference, sentimentality or, worse still, collusion with suffering. From this point of view, the doctor's position is analogous to that of the analyst, when he or she becomes aware of the destructive potentialities of his or her own emotions in countertransference (which is defined as the sum of the analyst's unconscious reactions to the person under analysis, and in particular to their transference). Empathy entails responsibilities, and this underlines the need for a space of support, consultation and psychological assistance to be available for doctors and nurses, too, with regard to these matters.

Even the way in which patients are touched – a gentle, confident contact rather than an abrupt, hesitant one – can make a big difference and be sufficient to calm them down. The nurse who is aware of this recreates, through empathic physical care, that link with the earth, with the Great Mother who nourishes and sustains, at a time when this resource can preserve the individual's psychic wholeness and reawaken his or her vitality.

This kind of dialogue – light, and open not only to emotional but also to imaginative content – can help to create a process in which patients rediscover a semblance of unitary signification and can differentiate from themselves the threatening unconscious content whose symbolic and cognitive value they can sense intuitively. This process almost always directly involves family members, whose physical and emotional closeness to the patient must, in my opinion, be actively encouraged, modulated and protected by those responsible for their treatment.

There is a subtle link between sadness and relief, between the thought-provoking experience of the limit on the one hand, and the gift of lightness on the other; between the condition of someone who has had personal experience of the thin thread on which life hangs, and the good humour of one who has recovered and who allows him-or herself the gift of smiling again. This link is never so clear as in the period after recovery from serious illness.

Time only is our own

Even when the soul imprisoned in a sick body longs for death because it has suffered too much, the body continues to resist; it possesses an enormous inertia, a formidable deterrent to letting itself die. Whenever I see men and women struck down by a pulmonary oedema or a massive heart attack, I am amazed at how the body invariably rebels, struggles, writhes, gesticulates and protests; the body always rejects its end, whatever the circumstances; it defends itself with every fibre, cell and nerve, even when it is old, until the last. Its mission is univocal, summed up in a single choice, made once and for all: it cannot but set its lymph against death. The afflicted body surges with every breath at its exuberance of life in a chorus of voices, organs, cells, molecules and quivers, until its final breath.[11] The artist Claudio Parmiggiani writes:

> Death. This is a rather delicate matter. In this connection I can only quote the words of my father's father, uttered when close to the final moment. I heard him say it myself: 'Death to death!', as a gesture of defiance and in regret at leaving this life.[12]

The psyche too is resistant to the prospect of death, of course – but this notion, the Stoics argued, derives from logic. For the psyche, death always comes without warning, because we cannot know its reality; like nothingness, it is not an object directly inherent in our psychic experience. All that is possible is a symbolic or metaphysical representation of it.

Epicurus wrote to his pupil and friend Maecenas:

> Accustom thyself to believe that death is nothing to us, for good and evil imply sentience, and death is the privation of all sentience; therefore a right understanding that death is nothing to us makes the mortality of life enjoyable, not by adding to life an illimitable time, but by taking away the yearning after immortality.[13]

However, it is the experience of pain and illness that reminds us, in life, of our mortal condition, and brings home to us the closeness of the boundary and of death itself. 'It is not because he falls ill that man dies; fundamentally, it is because he may die that man may fall ill,' says Foucault.[14] When it seems that life has already left the body, near the end, one waits until the flickering flame of that dying and still loved body goes out completely. Everything that has passed, that has been unique, once and for all, comes back to us: the people, the places, the atmospheres, the beauty, the tensions, the conflicts, 'echoes of footsteps in the memory', but also ruins and ancient presences, memories over which our steps still walk. If every day, from birth onwards, a new interval is spent, there is no day when life does not seek a way of affirming itself, of budding and blooming. There is no age limit to this: even the body of a centenarian, perhaps possessing a wonderful mind (even the most silent old people conceal hidden pearls of wisdom), deserves to be helped in this struggle by all possible means. From this point of view, the paradoxical quip 'death to death' is only too welcome.

No psychological determinism can hold out against the vital impulse of the body, in health or in sickness. Medicine, in the often one-sided pursuit of its mission for life, responds by every means possible to this natural propensity: with the help of technology it facilitates it and prolongs it, but, unfortunately, in so doing it commercializes itself. On the other hand, psychology may fall into thanatotropic determinism, where every somatic disease finds its psychological explanation; that every soul can seek, and perhaps create, the means of its own end may be true, but from this point of view it is completely insignificant. And meanwhile, like the doctors, psychologists sell themselves. Between these two extremes there may be a 'middle way'.

In this reductive sense, then, medicine and psychology are situated at opposite poles of the desire for omnipotence, human ambition and control. They stand on the 'physical' and 'mental' level respectively of the final goal, which remains unattainable, because it overcomes us and betrays us.

No one is better placed to know the nature of time than an old person close to death. The psychological unknowableness of death, especially at an advanced age, can enrich the perception of time, bestowing on the individual the gift of a love for life. Seneca wrote to his friend Lucilius:

> What man wilt thou show me that hath put any price upon time, that esteemeth of a day, and that understandeth that he daily dieth? For herein are we deceived, because we suppose death to be far off from us; and yet notwithstanding, the greater part thereof is already over-passed, and all our years that are behind, death holdeth in his possession. Do therefore, my Lucilius, that which, as thou writest unto me, thou doest: embrace and lay hold on each hour. So will it come to pass that thou shalt be less in suspense for tomorrow, if thou lay hold and fasten thy hands on today. Whiles life is deferred, it fleeteth. All other things, my Lucilius, are foreign to us; time only is our own.[15]

Life hanging by a thread

The word 'angina' has the same etymological origin as 'anxiety' and 'anguish' and the German *Angst*: the common root is Latin *angere* and Greek *ágkhein*, to squeeze or strangle; the Latin noun *angustiae* (*enge*, in German) means 'narrowness'.[16] *Angina pectoris* is constriction, a spasmodic condition, contraction, oppression. In literature, *Angst* is linked to the existential solitude of Western human beings, since the 'death of God' – individuals abandoned to their fate, facing the extreme solitude and the unease of their own disillusionment, though repaid by the benefits of 'civilization' and science. The modern human being is afflicted by a range of 'cardiovascular disease risk factors', the frequency of whose occurrence increases exponentially as soon as a country begins to develop economically. One in five deaths is linked to obesity.[17] The phrase 'risk factors' denotes an ability to increase the risk of cardiovascular events, such as heart attacks and strokes. Such factors can accelerate the development, and foment the spread and severity, of atherosclerotic disease at the level of all the vascular areas of the organism. In this sense, atherosclerosis may be likened to a particular inner predisposition of the organism to decline, for the most part predetermined at birth, and capable of interacting with numerous environmental factors. The process begins in childhood and involves the progressive or sudden remodelling of the arteries, which can result, at a more advanced age, in obstruction or closure, beginning with a thickened or diseased artery wall, either gradually or suddenly and unpredictably. The risk factors are arterial hypertension, hypercholesterolaemia, overweight, diabetes mellitus and behavioural factors such as smoking, a diet rich in sugar, animal fat and salt, and of course genetic predisposition. The appearance of the disease on the clinical level may be sudden, or the atherosclerosis may lead silently over a long period to an advanced condition of functional impairment of one or more vital organs, such as the heart, the brain and the kidneys. So there may be a sudden crisis, in the form of a heart attack, stroke or acute necrosis of the kidney tubules; or an insidious evolution towards chronic organ impairment; or a combination of both, where acute episodes are associated with a progressive, undulating loss of the organ's functionality. Of course the intensity of the disease is variable, on a continuous spectrum ranging from mild or transitory conditions to severe or persistent forms, and reflects a different propensity to illness. Atherosclerosis is like a planned death which undermines life from within, even though it is part of that life, causing the progressive degeneration of the vessels that nourish the various organs of the body, which, in acute or chronic ways, are forced into reduced activity and cell death.

Arterial hypertension, obesity and diabetes mellitus, but also the habit of smoking, depression and anxiety, are all characterized by adrenergic hyperactivity, a tipping of the balance between the two main antagonistic systems of the neurovegetative apparatus – the sympathetic nervous system and the vagus nerve – in favour of the adrenergic principle of stimulating the production of energy and activating it with respect to the environment. If sustained over time, this condition leads to a high-consumption and high-speed economy, particularly useful when outer conditions are difficult. One might conjecture that there has been a selection of this trait, to foster social adaptation. Adrenergic activation and the development of angst may coincide: the same mechanisms that are set in motion to promote adaptation to life and the dominance of the environment, if subjected to continual over-stimulation (as happens in modern mass societies) might cause unconscious emotional unease.

Adrenergic hypertonia and vascular atherosclerosis would therefore become the somatic reminder of a libidinal energy withdrawn from itself and invested in the outer world. The disease of the body would in this way compensate for the imperialistic and expansionistic hubris of the risk factors, of the psychic bulimia which underlies them and which, crossing the threshold of environmental adaptation, has confused the will to power with the survival instinct. The individual will enter into the parabola of unlimited consumption, like a sort of compensated drug addict, who alternates the search for pleasure through consumption with the protected but uncritical world whose variables the person thinks he or she can control, thanks to a construction based on the clarity and order of rationalism, and on the technological transformation of the environment. In this way the appearance of the somatic disease exercises a compensation, starting from the body, against the one-sidedness typical of the first half of life or the self-imposed prison of overwork, overeating and hyperconsumption. The risk factors are the first sign, the premonitory announcement. In this context, illness has a depressive effect, which, however, is in fact compensatory with respect to the excesses of the collective function-alist frenzy. For we only use antihypertensive, antidiabetic and lipid-lowering drugs; we do not realize that a possible solution might lie in renouncing one-sidedness, recognizing the importance of listening to a voice which is not that of the ego and which expresses itself through the body. This deceleration is a first step, a deceleration which is not apotropaic, but conscious of the one-sided attitude; it is a departure from the customary patterns and dominant attitudes, giving the individual time for quiet reflection.

Many people suffer a heart attack or stroke soon after they retire, having silently borne the burden of their own Chronos-dominated time, of a whole life devoted to the rhythms of work and consumption. People with a large somatic heart, a heart full of scars, repeated infarctions and repressed sad-ness. As Hillman points out, the term 'infarction' (from the Latin *farctus*, stuffed, filled) may represent the heart stuffed by its own images which have not gone out into circulation, of a person's unlived lives, which will be inher-ited by their children, as burdens of the exile of the imagination.

The limit may come with advanced age and exclusion from functional society, which does not recognize the old person's qualities, such as wisdom and concision – while the old risk becoming depressed, if they have interior-ized the values of youth culture. How many elderly heart patients, once slim and active, highly strung and energetic, are left weak by heart failure, by an organism debilitated by the insufficient nutrition of the tissues, by the slow-ing flow of blood through its vessels, and are forced to reduce all activity. Great old people in whom it is hard to fish life out of the deep waters of depression. Once again it will be the soma that materializes the 'Dionysiac' in the dampness of water retention, in the oedemas that swell heart patients' extremities and faces at an advanced stage of their illness, and which will also swell their stomach, taking away their appetite. They are sometimes abandoned to the functional, aseptic embrace of a nursing home.

Think, too, of the epidemic of senile dementia, that degeneration of the higher cerebral functions, which, once the cognitive function has been dam-aged badly enough (with the thinning of the cortical grey matter and the widening of the cerebral sulci), will reassert the re-emerging animal emo-tionality, often hitherto denied or unexpressed, which is rediscovered in its fullness and richness, through the experience of forced attendance and sad-ness, on the part of the relatives. It is not unusual for people to become attached with previously unknown intensity to a parent suffering from Alzheimer's disease or vascular dementia.

Figure 7.2 shows the angiograms of two patients with ACS (acute coronary syndrome). Visibly, the calibre of the artery is reduced for a short length to a fraction of a millimetre. Just as the seemingly heavy matter is supported by

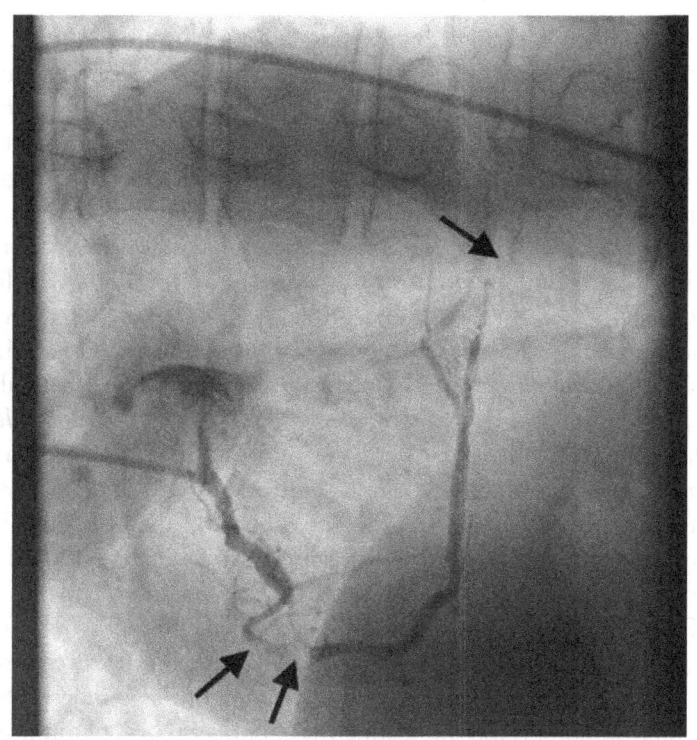

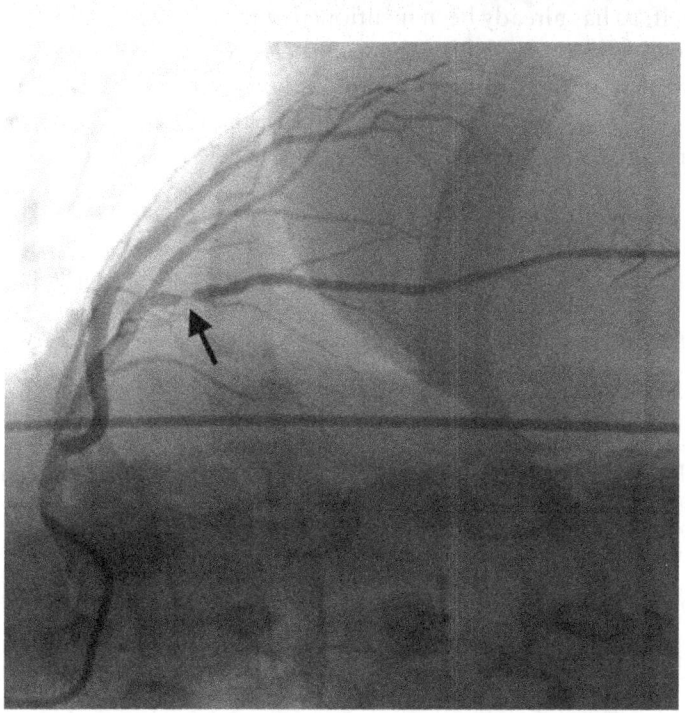

Figure 7.2 Two coronary angiograms in two different patients with acute coronary syndrome. Left side: left anterior descending branch of the left coronary artery. Right side: right coronary artery. The arrows indicate severe blockages.

Author's own illustrations.

the lightness of a multitude of invisible corpuscles, connected by numerous minute forces and subtle signals, so life, seemingly stable and concrete, and linked to the immediate perception of one's body, hangs by a hair, a thin thread without which it would be snuffed out, like an electric light at the flick of a switch. As can be seen from the illustration, which shows angiograms of two patients who have suffered acute myocardial infarction, it may literally be a tiny trickle of blood. Looking at such images and the patients from whom they were taken, one thinks of how the body, for all its stability and symmetry, is supported by the imperceptible, the unpredictable and the ineffable. Behind these thin threads we may sense the closeness of God – that God who in Islam says to humankind: 'We are closer to him than his jugular vein' (Quran, L, 16). One is struck, therefore, by the saying '*Allah muqallib al qulub*' – Allah is he who 'mixes' or 'overturns' hearts. Curiously, the words 'to mix' (*qallaba*), and the reflexive form 'to be overturned' (*inqalaba*), are both derived from the word 'heart' (*qalb*). The infarction may therefore be derived symbolically not just from the occlusion of a coronary artery, but from the fact of the heart being crammed with its own images. Once the circular action of mixing the vital substance of being, which embraces the whole of psychic life, ceases, the images are no longer able to get out. Desire comes from an environment external to the ego; not betraying one's own desire but understanding its command is like subjecting the ego to a process of initiation which is life itself; as has already been mentioned with reference to alchemical metallurgy, it will be beaten, shaped, bent and cleaned in the flames of the desire to know the face of the other, before assuming the form that will give it its value. The 'cure' might therefore lie in rediscovering the courage to desire and to 'see' through desire; in making the heart's surface purer.

Notes

1 Biagi 1971. Interview conducted in 1971 but first shown only after the author's death in 1975. Part of the exchange quoted in the text is available in a short YouTube recording of a fragment of the interview: www.youtube.com/watch?v=KtrCfC2r 798 Accessed 30th October 2017.
2 Nietzsche 1882, aphorism 125 (The Madman), pp. 79–80.
3 According to Hisdosus Scholasticus's commentary on Calcidius, Heraclitus compared the soul to a spider which rushes to any part of its web when it is damaged by a fly, as if she suffered until the body's wound is repaired. The soul is described as '*firme et proportionaliter iuncta*' to the body; the idea of proportion is appropriate to Heraclitus. The swift movement of the spider starting from the heart or centre of the web can also be seen as an ancient understanding of the neurovegetative tensions in parts of the body or damaged organs. See Heraclitus, Fragment D 67a, p. 289 (M. 115, p. 576 ff.).
4 Zoja 2003, pp. 190–191.
5 World Health Organization (WHO) 2004, Figure 27, p. 51.
6 Weinert 2008.

7 Kalsched 1996, pp. 37–38.
8 The word numinous, from the Latin *numinosus*, indicates the character of other-ness, which as such is the basis of the possible experience of otherness itself.
9 Jung 1954, pp. 244–245.
10 Borgna 2009, p. 35.
11 Note for health professionals. Massive adrenergic stimulation in acute somatic stress differs from the sympathetic reactions shown in struggling or trying to escape, since it is determined by intense afferent reflex activation of the cardiovascular apparatus. The reflex arch is triggered by the suffering vital somatic organs; hence the central nervous system is not primarily activated. Psychic numbing mediated by peripheral vagal reflexes in acute cardio-respiratory diseases can also occur, often transiently, and is associated with variable degrees of hemodynamic compromise. In contrast, the activation of the central dorsolateral vagal complex, that is responsible for freezing in psychic trauma when it becomes inescapable (as when an animal prey is captured by its predator and all its attempts to escape fail), appears to be a central phenomenon. Thus the complex and variable interactions in response to psychological trauma, with its neo-cortical, lymbic and basal brain components, in the context of exogenous threat or harm, appear to constitute a different phenom-enology from that of endogenous acute systemic disease (see Ogden et al. 2006).
12 Parmiggiani 1995, p. 25.
13 Laertius, p. 652.
14 Foucault 1963, p. 191.
15 Seneca, p. 167 (Epist. 1, 1).
16 Freud 1915–17, p. 342, for a discussion of the etymology and its significance:

> I avoid entering upon a discussion as to whether our language means the same or distinct things by the words anxiety, fear or fright. I think that anxiety is used in connection with a condition regardless of any objective, while fear is essentially directed toward an object. Fright, on the other hand, seems really to possess a special meaning, which emphasizes the effects of a danger which is precipitated without any expectance or readiness of fear. Thus we might say that anxiety protects man from fright.

He goes on to say, p. 343:

> We believe we know the early impression which the emotion of fear repeats. We think it is birth itself which combines that complex of painful feelings, of a discharge of impulses, of physical sensations, which has become the prototype for the effect of danger to life, and is ever after repeated within us as a condition of fear. The tremendous heightening of irritability through the interruption of the circulation (internal respiration) was at the time the cause of the experience of fear; the first fear was therefore toxic. The name anxiety – angustial – narrowness, emphasizes the characteristic tightening of the breath, which was at the time a consequence of an actual situation and is henceforth repeated almost regularly in the emotion. We shall also recognize how significant it is that this first condition of fear appeared dur-ing the separation from the mother.

17 Masters 2013.

Bibliography

Biagi, Enzo (1971), Interview with Pierpaolo Pasolini for the Rai Television Programme 'Terza B: Facciamo L'appello'. www.teche.rai.it/2017/03/enzo-biagi-e-pierpaolo-pasolini-un-confronto. For an account of the interview by Biagi, see www.lucaniain rete.it/rubriche/Interviste/Pasolini%20intervista%20esclusiva%20di%20Enzo%20 Biagi.html. Both websites accessed 30th October 2017.

Borgna, Eugenio (2009), *Le Emozioni Ferite. Wounded Emotions*, Milan: Feltrinelli, 2009.

British Museum, 'Frame 3, Episodes in Hunefer's Judgement, 19th Dynasty, c. 1280 BC', from the Book of the Dead of Hunefer. www.britishmuseum.org/research/ collection_online/collection_object_details.aspx?objectId=114851&partId=1&se archText=weighing+of+the+heart&page=1 Accessed 30th October 2017.

Foucault, Michel (1963), *Naissance de la clinique. The Birth of the Clinic: An Archaeology of Medical Perception*, translated by Alan Mark Sheridan, London & New York: Routledge, 1989 [c. 1973].

Freud, Sigmund (1915–17), *Vorlesungen zur Einführung in die Psychoanalyse. A General Introduction to Psychoanalysis*, Lecture 25, 'General Theory of the Neuroses', translated by Stanley Hall, Mansfield Centre, CT: Martino Publishing, 2009.

Heraclitus, *The Art and Thought of Heraclitus: An Edition of the Fragments with Translation and Commentary*, by Charles H. Hahn, Cambridge: Cambridge University Press, 1979.

Jung, Carl Gustav (1954), *Praxis der Psychotherapie. The Practice of Psychotherapy: Essays on the Psychology of Transference and Other Subjects*, Bollingen Series XX, Vol. 16 of the Collected Works of C.G. Jung, translated by Richard Francis Carrington Hull, Princeton, NJ: Princeton University Press, 1966.

Kalsched, Donald (1996), *The Inner World of Trauma: Archetypal Defences of the Personal Spirit*, London: Routledge, 1996.

Laertius, Diogenes, *Lives of Eminent Philosophers*, translated by Robert Drew Hicks, Vol. 2, 1925 The Loeb Classical Library, London: William Heineman, 1925.

Masters, Ryan K. et al. (2013), 'The Impact of Obesity on US Mortality Levels: The Importance of Age and Cohort Factors in Population Estimates', *American Journal of Public Health*, 103, part 10 (2013), pp. 1895–1901.

Nietzsche, Friedrich (1882), *Die Fröhliche Wissenschaft. The Gay Science*, translated by Thomas Common, Overland Park, KS: Digireads, 2009.

Ogden, Pat et al. (2006), *Trauma and the Body: A Sensory-Motor Approach to Psychotherapy*, New York: W.W. Norton & Co., 2006.

Parmiggiani, Claudio (1995), *Stella, sangue, spirito*, Parma: Pratiche Editrice, 1995.

Seneca, Lucius Annaeus, *Ad Lucilium Epistulae Morales*, The Works of Lucius Annaeus Seneca, newly inlarged and corrected by Thomas Lodge, London: William Stansby, 1620 [c.1614].

Weinert, Craig R. & Sprenkle, Mark (2008), 'Post-ICU Consequences of Patient Wakefulness and Sedative Exposure during Mechanical Ventilation', *Intensive Care Medicine*, 34 (2008), pp. 82–90.

World Health Organization (2004), *The Global Burden of Disease*, 2004 update, Geneva, Switzerland: WHO Press.

Zoja, Luigi (2003), *Storia dell'Arroganza: Psicologia e Limiti dello Sviluppo. Growth and Guilt: Psychology and the Limits of Development*, translated by Henry Martin, London: Routledge, 1995.

Chapter 8

The globalization of medicine

Towards an ecological medicine

The functionalism and the nihilism intrinsic to the age of technology might be linked to the exploitation of the emotional, though biological, effect of centuries of undernourishment and privation. An obvious example is the epidemic of obesity and cardiovascular risk factors in the developing countries, which, as soon as they begin to grow, assimilate the consumeristic, debt-based model. Eric Hobsbawm helps to explain the founding myth of this kind of phenomenon:

> The ideologists of the late twentieth century preferred to abandon the task of pursuing reason and social change, leaving them to the automatic operations of a world of purely rational individuals, allegedly maximising their benefits through a rationally operating market that naturally tended, when free of outside interference, towards a lasting equilibrium.[1]

The implications for medicine are clear, especially if one considers the unsustainable expansion of the superfluous in this model of socioeconomic development. Processes which took centuries to be completed in Europe are today condensed into a few decades in most parts of the world, which leads to cultural impoverishment associated with an explosive demography. There is an institutionalization of 'culture' as a uniquely rational heritage, whose references continue to be predominantly western. Science alone seems to dominate the theatre of knowledge. Its power to transform reality is paramount. At the same time, the structure of reality is transferred to the powerful sphere of virtual flows, and that makes it difficult for the individual to develop an ethic of responsibility. Doctors who accept the indications of the 'market' without differentiation, who do not oppose the superfluous, are bound to be successful, for they will reconcile the power of the flows (and their global influences) with the (limited) power of their own experience (whose influences are local). Doctors who oppose the superfluous, on the other hand, will come up against insurmountable obstacles, unless they propose a different vision of the meaning and speed of science, from within science itself. An ecology of medicine considers the need to change the mental borders of the doctor's actions in the context of science, and takes into account a slow pace, that of the whole planet. It has more respect for the life of *physis* in preserving the individual's life, doing everything possible to reconcile the two aspects of the vision human beings have of themselves and the use they want to make of science.

There is great ethical significance in the fact that, as a result of its transformation into a show, the language of emotion is often devalued today. The universe of feeling, its language and its complexity, are no longer distinguished from unreflecting emotionalism or from drive, with serious consequences on the cognitive and moral levels; alternatively, feeling is often confused with its surrogates, with mental representation. The difference between thought and feeling is well expressed by Eugenio Borgna, when he writes:

> The emotions say what is going on in us, in our psyche, in our inner world, in our soul; but the emotions are (also) carriers of knowledge: of a knowledge which pulls us into the heart of some life experiences that our rational knowledge cannot reach.[2]

The separation between the two levels and the loss of a vocabulary of emotion have been accentuated by the extreme acceleration of technological development, and consequently of the historical processes.

The relativization of every ethic of conviction (also known as an ethic of principle) by the great cognitive apparatus of science could come into conflict with an absolute faith which survives within science itself, an intimate, structural conviction that objectifying reason is preferable to any other form of knowledge. As Nietzsche said, it is far from being a neutral faith on the moral level. Hidden in this tendency, he maintained, there is a 'destructive principle, hostile to life. "Will to Truth" – that might be a concealed Will to Death', which thus affirms a world different from that of life and can only propose a negative idea of freedom.[3] Pasolini said: 'In order to love tradition you must have a great love for life. The bourgeoisie doesn't love life, it owns it. And this implies a lack of respect for a tradition understood as a tradition of privilege and inherited status.'[4]

Today, in the world of the online society, every ethic of responsibility[5] is forced to become truly complex, and to develop global references and think of the fortunes of its own group as if it were the whole of humanity; otherwise it will run the risk of becoming 'relativized' in its turn, unable to withstand the test of singularities. A fundamental obstacle is presented by the economic dogmas of exclusion. Exclusion from the web today means total economic marginality, exclusion from participation in the productive systems revolutionized by information technology, which still remains alien to a significant proportion of the inhabitants of the planet, who have become the shadow of the consumer society, having struggled to survive the end of the traditional world and having become in their turn the prey of dangerous Narcissistic postmodern temptations, namely the present-day forms of fanaticism.

It is belonging to the techno-capitalist sphere that gives one the right to citizenship; this is tantamount to saying that the more one conforms to the power of technocracy, *even by simply being able to access its services*, the more confident one may be that one's own human rights will be guaranteed. The prize for citizenship is morally problematic, for it is based on exclusivity and market competition. Ethical universality is never granted, since property norms are disproportionately pre-eminent over human rights: this fundamental split tends to remain unmentioned, unelaborated and therefore veiled – like a pre-conscious, shameful, naked truth. The increasing undesirability of human rights is linked to the defence of the prize of citizenship. The otherness of the other and the other's humanity become irrelevant, especially for competitors, in the face of the issue of re- or de-territorialisation. Rights have become a matter not of principle, but of economic development. Thus, the hegemony of patrimonial norms increasingly prioritizes the need for defence of geographically acquired citizenship advantages, reducing the issue of human rights to an irritating thorn in the flesh, especially for those belonging to the lower classes of richer societies. Security is progressively based on an immunizing paradigm combined with the crisis of the Subject.

For medicine, the question remains whether this predominance of a very questionable 'reason' does not obstruct the consideration of the patient as a fellow human being, as a person who is close to us on an emotional and symbolic level; whether we risk continuing to mistake the part for the whole, to exclude the mystery of the other in a systematic manner. Nihilism, the will to death of science, would be realized in life, by reaffirming the death that is denied in another way – in relational impoverishment, moral indifference and a lack of respect for the environment. Hence, this respect should extend beyond the human sphere, to include what Chiron symbolized in his chimerical nature: the rich diversity of the animal and plant worlds. The other creatures on the planet should be considered as 'kin', sharing the same destiny as us on a damaged earth. A renewed sense of intimacy with the animal world – but also with plants, forests, mountains, rivers and seas (the 'ecosystem', the earth) – proves to be a radical limitation of human one-sidedness, a renewed sense of presence to oneself, beyond the limits of anthropocentrism. Living on this earth together with the great variety of other individual beings in the *physis* requires us to develop, or regain, a capacity to relate to death, grief and mourning.[6] The background noise of functionalism is heard by all; it forces us into hurrying, for fear of not being able to keep up. Freud stated in *Civilization and Its Discontents* that 'we will not forget that present-day man does not feel happy in his God-like character.'[7]

Science, by formulating a rational discourse, sets its own limit, which is also that of its own falsifiability. Without the rational limit there can be no transcending of thought by those who follow it, and the will to truth risks becoming a 'truth neurosis'. The problem is rendering the use we make of science falsifiable too, that is, trying not to submit passively to its (irrational) force which moves history. This makes many hope for an age of great transition, of a transformation of language and of the human imagination. While humankind goes through a phase of great expansion of rational knowledge and the consolidation of the power to do things, it still has confidence, strengthened by the improvements in the living conditions of postmodern humans, in its capacity for learning and for adaptation/correction. But life, and therefore nature and history, is impoverished and distorted by the denial of that which psychologically regenerates it, namely natural death. The container no longer has sufficient eschatological significance. And all over the globe, history seems to have been impoverished, as if it were being narrated by a single victor: advanced capitalism, with its commodification of all forms of life, and of life itself. It is not surprising that people in this age are losing interest in the obsession with thought and content, asking insistently for silence, perhaps sensing the imminent preponderance of form, of the ethical need for a continual reduction of weight. For the time being we have fallen into the trap of narcissism and entertainment.

'There is always war,' as Mordo Nahum says in Primo Levi's *The Truce*, but, unlike his work ethic, where work is conceived of as 'everything, and only that, which leads to profit without limiting freedom',[8] the ethic has shifted from work to profit and has replaced the myth of positive freedom with that of the uniformity of affluence. Nothing can escape the metaphysical abyss of the globalized market of the web, until the ancient container – the earth – will cease to appear infinite (*titanism* as an element of the maternal; it should be remembered that Prometheus was a Titan). This will go on for as long as the new container can continue to exist – the container of a hyper(ir)rational faith in the power of technology and, only through it, in the power of the human will.

But this container is already shaky. For:

> Subjective anxieties combine with a general disquiet, and private unease cannot be separated from the unease of civilization. The contemporary world no longer moves along the line of Leopardi's 'magnificent progressive destinies', but sees progress as a possibility of decline and expansion as extinction. But what rule can we apply to growth, how can we always exactly find the right measure? It is possible that what technology has constructed may be preserved if it is reinterpreted in a higher reason, where growth curves into the boundary and can be revived only by turning back. But here it is as well to keep silent about this possible wisdom, pointing out, however, that human beings come to measure through pain, for in pain they discover the extent of their own finiteness. For where feeling is intense, suffering is unavoidable, and joy can be possessed only through the knowledge of pain. What is certain, at any rate, is the fact that the stage on which pain performs today is the ambiguity of power.[9]

Contemporary medicine already contains the seeds of profound change, which is beginning to appear together with the effects of social and environmental unsustainability. Although it is possible that technology will find some solutions in the future, today no one can deny the extent and irreversibility of the destruction that is occurring, with a vigorous spread of regressive phenomena, after the fall of the traditional world. The abuses of the patriarchy are most frequently replaced by the abuses of the society of brothers, of regression to the pre-paternal male, equipped with technological media and reductive, in contrast to a more desirable openness to the values of the feminine world, which have been described in various parts of this book. The competitiveness of the economic system seems to reinforce this tendency and to foment a paradoxical masculinization of women in the world of work.

However, this inertia of history and the ethical degeneration that derives from it are opposed by an increasing number of initiatives open to a language founded on listening to others, on memory and on complexity – of which this book aims to be one of many examples.

What is proposed here is also another form of courage: that of overturning thought from the invisible and interior immanence of consciousness, of self-reflective reason, to an even more invisible and intuitive immanence of the language of the heart. Human beings, in daring to go beyond the needs of the protective container of reason, which has replaced God while insatiably absorbing his omnipotence towards technology, risk life itself by a hair's breadth, by overcoming (with the courage to embrace it) the alien nature of all that is dearest and most paradoxical to them, such as love, pain, childhood, ancestry, nature and death.

This act requires an abandonment of the reductive position of functionalism, and of self-referential humanism, in favour of the development of a different image of humankind with respect to the conditionings of *techne*.

Notes

1 Hobsbawm 2013, p. 198.
2 Borgna 2009, p. 14.
3 Nietzsche 1882, Aphorism 344, p. 132.
4 Pasolini 1962.
5 Weber 1919, pp. 120–122.
6 Haraway 2016, chapter 4: 'Making Kin, Anthropocene, Capitalocene, Plantationocene, Chthulucene', pp. 99–103.
7 The assertion comes at the end of the following passage:

> These things that, by his science and technology, man has brought about on this earth, on which he first appeared as a feeble animal organism and on which each individual of his species must once more make its entry ('oh inch of nature!') as a helpless suckling-these things do not only sound like a fairy tale, they are an actual fulfilment of every – or of almost every – fairytale wish. All these assets he may lay claim to as his cultural acquisition. Long ago he formed an ideal conception of omnipotence and omniscience which he embodied in his gods. To these gods he attributed everything that seemed unattainable to his wishes, or that was forbidden to him. One may say, therefore, that these gods were cultural ideals. Today he has come very close to the attainment of this ideal, he has almost become a god himself. Only, it is true, in the fashion in which ideals are usually attained according to the general judgement of humanity. Not completely; in some respects not at all, in others only half way. Man has, as it were, become a kind of prosthetic God. When he puts on all his auxiliary organs he is truly magnificent; but those organs have not grown on to him and they still give him much trouble at times. Nevertheless, he is entitled to console himself with the thought that this development will come to an end precisely with the year 1930 A.D. Future ages will bring with them new and probably unimaginably great advances in this field of civilization and will increase man's likeness to God still more. But in the interests of our investigations, we will not forget that present-day man does not feel happy in his Godlike character.
>
> (Freud 1929, pp. 37–39)

8 Levi 1961–62, pp. 57, 51.
9 Natoli 1986, p. 384.

Bibliography

Borgna, Eugenio (2009), *Le Emozioni Ferite*, Milan: Feltrinelli, 2009.
Freud, Sigmund (1929), *Das Unbehagen in der Kultur. Civilization and Its Discontents* (1930), translated by James Strachey, *The Standard Edition of the Complete*

Psychological Works of Sigmund Freud, Vol. XXI (1927–1931) published as a single volume, New York: Norton, 1961.

Haraway, Donna (2016), *Staying with the Trouble: Making Kin in the Chthulucene*, Durham, NC: Duke University Press, 2016.

Hobsbawm, Eric (2013), 'The Intellectuals: Role, Function and Paradox', in *Fractured Times: Culture and Society in the Twentieth Century*, London: Little, Brown, 2013.

Levi, Primo (1961–62), *La Tregua*, Turin: Einaudi, 1997.

Natoli, Salvatore (1986), *L'esperienza del Dolore: Le Forme del Patire nella Cultura Occidentale. The Experience of Pain: The Forms of Suffering in Western Culture*, Milan: Feltrinelli, 2008.

Nietzsche, Friedrich (1882), *Die Fröhliche Wissenschaft. The Gay Science*, translated by Thomas Common, Overland Park, KS: Digireads, 2009.

Pasolini, Pier Paolo (1962), 'Risposta a un Insoddisfatto', *Vie Nuove*, 22 November, 1962.

Weber, Max (1919), 'Politik als Beruf', in *Gesammelte Politische Schriften*, Munich, 1921, pp. 396–450, [originally a speech at Munich University, 1918, published in 1919 by Duncker & Humblodt, Munich]. 'Politics as a Vocation', in *From Max Weber: Essays in Sociology*, translated, edited and with an introduction by Hans Heinrich Gerth and Charles Wright Mills, London: Routledge, 1948.

Index

Note: Page numbers for figures are in italics.